Ergebnisse der Anatomie und Entwicklungsgeschichte
Advances in Anatomy, Embryology and Cell Biology
Revues d'anatomie et de morphologie expérimentale
Springer-Verlag Berlin Heidelberg New York

This journal publishes reviews and critical articles covering the entire field of normal anatomy (cytology, histology, cyto- and histochemistry, electron microscopy, macroscopy, experimental morphology and embryology and comparative anatomy). Papers dealing with anthropology and clinical morphology will also be accepted with the aim of encouraging co-operation between anatomy and related disciplines.

Papers, which may be in English, French or German, are normally commissioned, but original papers and communications may be submitted and will be considered so long as they deal with a subject comprehensively and meet the requirements of the Ergebnisse.

For speed of publication and breadth of distribution, this journal appears in single issues which can be purchased separately; 6 issues constitute one volume.

It is a fundamental condition that manuscripts submitted should not have been published elsewhere, in this or any other country, and the author must undertake not to publish elsewhere at a later date.

25 copies of each paper are supplied free of charge.

Les résultats publient des sommaires et des articles critiques concernant l'ensemble du domaine de l'anatomie normale (cytologie, histologie, cyto et histochimie, microscopie électronique, macroscopie, morphologie expérimentale, embryologie et anatomie comparée. Seront publiés en outre les articles traitant de l'anthropologie et de la morphologie clinique, en vue d'encourager la collaboration entre l'anatomie et les disciplines voisines.

Seront publiés en priorité les articles expressément demandés nous tiendrons toutefois compte des articles qui nous seront envoyés dans la mesure où ils traitent d'un sujet dans son ensemble et correspondent aux standards des «Résultats». Les publications seront faites en langues anglaise, allemande et française.

Dans l'intérêt d'une publication rapide et d'une large diffusion les travaux publiés paraitront dans des cahiers individuels, diffusés séparément: 6 cahiers forment un volume.

En principe, seuls les manuscrits qui n'ont encore été publiés ni dans le pays d'origine ni à l'étranger peuvent nous être soumis. L'auteur d'engage en outre à ne pas les publier ailleurs ultérieurement.

Les auteurs recevront 25 exemplaires gratuits de leur publication.

Die Ergebnisse dienen der Veröffentlichung zusammenfassender und kritischer Artikel aus dem Gesamtgebiet der normalen Anatomie (Cytologie, Histologie, Cyto- und Histochemie, Elektronenmikroskopie, Makroskopie, experimentelle Morphologie und Embryologie und vergleichende Anatomie). Aufgenommen werden ferner Arbeiten anthropologischen und morphologisch-klinischen Inhaltes, mit dem Ziel die Zusammenarbeit zwischen Anatomie und Nachbardisziplinen zu fördern.

Zur Veröffentlichung gelangen in erster Linie angeforderte Manuskripte, jedoch werden auch eingesandte Arbeiten und Originalmitteilungen berücksichtigt, sofern sie ein Gebiet umfassend abhandeln und den Anforderungen der ,, Ergebnisse" genügen. Die Veröffentlichungen erfolgen in englischer, deutscher oder französischer Sprache.

Die Arbeiten erscheinen im Interesse einer raschen Veröffentlichung und einer weiten Verbreitung als einzeln berechnete Hefte; je 6 Hefte bilden einen Band.

Grundsätzlich dürfen nur Manuskripte eingesandt werden, die vorher weder im Inland noch im Ausland veröffentlicht worden sind. Der Autor verpflichtet sich, sie auch nachträglich nicht an anderen Stellen zu publizieren.

Die Mitarbeiter erhalten von ihren Arbeiten zusammen 25 Freiexemplare.

Manuscripts should be addressed to/Envoyer les manuscrits à/Manuskripte sind zu senden an:

Prof. Dr. A. BRODAL, Universitetet i Oslo, Anatomisk Institutt, Karl Johans Gate 47 (Domus Media), Oslo 1/Norwegen.

Prof. W. HILD, Department of Anatomy, The University of Texas Medical Branch, Galveston, Texas 77550 (USA).

Prof. Dr. R. ORTMANN, Anatomisches Institut der Universität, 5 Köln-Lindenthal, Lindenburg.

Prof. Dr. T.H. SCHIEBLER, Anatomisches Institut der Universität, Koellikerstraße 6, 87 Würzburg.

Prof. Dr. G. TÖNDURY, Direktion der Anatomie, Gloriastraße 19, CH-8006 Zürich.

Prof. Dr. E. WOLFF, Collège de France, Laboratoire d'Embryologie Expérimentale, 49 bis Avenue de la belle Gabrielle, Nogent-sur-Marne 94/France.

Ergebnisse der Anatomie und Entwicklungsgeschichte
Advances in Anatomy, Embryology and Cell Biology
Revues d'anatomie et de morphologie expérimentale

45 · 1

Editores
A. Brodal, Oslo · W. Hild, Galveston · R. Ortmann, Köln
T. H. Schiebler, Würzburg · G. Töndury, Zürich · E. Wolff, Paris

J. Kartenbeck, H. Zentgraf
U. Scheer, W. W. Franke

The Nuclear Envelope
in Freeze-Etching

with 47 Figures

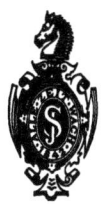

Springer-Verlag Berlin Heidelberg GmbH 1971

J. Kartenbeck, H. Zentgraf,

Dr. U. Scheer, Doz. Dr. W. W. Franke

Department of Cell Biology, Institute of

Biology II, University of Freiburg i. Br.,

D-7800 Freiburg/Germany, Schänzlestr. 9—15

ISBN 978-3-540-05538-9   ISBN 978-3-662-10390-6 (eBook)
DOI 10.1007/978-3-662-10390-6

Contents

Introduction

During the past twenty years the structure of the nuclear envelope, and in particular, that of its most distinct elements, the nuclear pore complexes, has been described from thin section electron microscopy (e.g., Brettschneider, 1952; Hartmann, 1953; Bahr and Beermann, 1954; Watson, 1954; Kautz and de Marsh, 1955; Watson, 1955), from metal-shadowed (e.g., Callan and Tomlin, 1950; Gall, 1954, 1956) and negatively stained (e.g., Franke, 1966, 1967; Gall, 1967; Yoo and Bayley, 1967) preparations of isolated nuclear membranes as revealing characteristics common to eukaryotic cells in general (recently reviewed, e.g., in Gouranton, 1969; Stevens and Andre, 1969; Franke, 1970).

In the recent years the freeze-etch technique (Steere, 1957) has proved to be a particularly useful tool in studying membraneous structures (e.g., Moor and Mühlethaler, 1963; Branton and Moor, 1964; Branton, 1966; Koehler, 1968b; Staehelin, 1968a; Northcote, 1968a; Branton, 1969; Moor, 1969a). So this method has especially broadened the knowledge, e.g., on bacterial membranes (Bayer and Remsen, 1970; Nanninga, 1970), on erythrocyte plasma membranes (Weinstein and Bullivant, 1967; Meyer and Winkelmann, 1970; da Silva and Branton, 1970; Tillack and Marchesi, 1970), on liver cell membranes (Chalcroft and Bullivant, 1970), on Golgi membranes (Werz and Kellner, 1970; Staehelin and Kiermayer, 1970), on synaptic vesicles (Moor et al., 1969), on retinal segments (Clark and Branton, 1968), on mitochondrial membranes (Keyhani and Kriz, 1969; Ruska and Ruska, 1969), on myelin sheath (Bischoff and Moor, 1967), on the thylakoid membranes of bacteria and plants (Giesbrecht and Drews, 1966; Park and Pfeifhofer, 1969a; Arntzen et al., 1969), on the plant cell tonoplast (Fineran, 1970a) and lysosomes (Matile, 1968) and on gas-vacuole membranes of Halobacterium (Stoeckenius and Kunau, 1968) and blue-green alga (Waaland and Branton, 1969; Jost and Jones, 1970).

Although sporadic remarks on nuclear envelope architectural details have been made in various freeze-etch studies (e.g., Moor and Mühlethaler, 1963; Branton and Moor, 1964; Leak, 1968; Koehler, 1968; Northcote and Lewis, 1968; Bishop, 1969; Allen and Hess, 1969; Bertaud et al., 1970; Bererhi and Malkani, 1970; Keyhani, 1970; Kouri et al., 1970; Neushul, 1970; Roberts and Northcote, 1970; Speth and Wunderlich, 1970; Wecke and Giesbrecht, 1970) no basic investigation has hitherto been made to compare the freeze-etch appearance of the nuclear envelopes of different cell types as, e.g., in order to examine whether there are universal structural principles at the freeze-etch level, too. Another question is whether special structural differences can be observed with the use of this technique, which is basically different from the other electron microscopic prepararations and, theoretically has a couple of advantages in terms of fixation and avoiding any dehydration procedures.

It appears to be necessary in the author's opinion to attract the general criticism of the reader to articles dealing with results of freeze-etch studies. In contrast to those investigations in which the biological material has been adapted in vivo to a glycerol environment (e.g., Moor and Mühlethaler, 1963; Branton and Moor, 1964; Moor, 1964; Branton, 1966; Giesbrecht and Drews, 1966; Hess, 1968; Northcote and Lewis, 1968; Fineran, 1970b) there are many examples in the literature in which the agent preventing ice crystal formation ("anti-freeze agent") has been applied using an inadequate way of preparation: So, for instance, some authors have put the living cells into a solution of, e.g., glycerol up to several hours prior to deep-freezing without checking their viability or even considering the possibility that the cells in questions could have been damaged or were already dead at the moment of freezing (e.g., Bauer, 1968; Fill and Branton, 1969; Nickel and Grieshaber, 1969; Plattner et al., 1969; Ruska and Ruska, 1969; Waaland and Branton, 1969; Bererhi and Malkani, 1970; Schwelitz et al., 1970; Speth and Wunderlich, 1970; Spycher, 1970; Tauschel and Speth, 1970; Weinstein et al., 1970; Wisse, 1970). Beyond that, Reith (1971) has recently demonstrated a considerable number of artifacts in the glycerol treatment as such, in particular those which are caused by the extraction of proteinaceous material Richter and Sleytr (1971) recently also attracted the attention to the possibility of lipid extraction during the freeze-preparation. Another source of misinterpretation of freeze-etching results comes from the hazardous discussion of results obtained with material that had been prestabilized with aldehydes, as representing so-called "in vivo structures" in the sense of the widely liked extreme extrapolation from the results of Moor (1964) and Hess (1968) obtained from non-fixed living fungal cells. On the other hand, in those experiments in which the cells had been adjusted to the anti-freeze agents, it cannot be a priori assumed that a specific result obtained refers to the non-adapted physiological state[1]. So, particular support for interpreting basic structural phenomena of frozen-etched cells should come from objects which can be rapidly frozen without the use of anti-freeze agents (e.g., Remsen and Lundgreen, 1966; Branton and Southworth, 1967; Branton et al., 1967; Sleytr et al., 1967, 1968; Meyer and Winkelmann, 1969; Brown et al., 1970; DaSilva and Branton, 1970; Neushul, 1970; Van Gool et al., 1970; Werz and Kellner, 1970; Brown and Franke, 1971).

A series of recent studies has contributed to the current concept of the nuclear membrane as being a cytomembrane with a peculiar character. It is characterized by an extremely low phospholipid: protein ratio (e.g., Berezney et al., 1970; Franke et al., 1970). In addition to many membrane characteristics which it shares with its most closely related membrane system, the rough endoplasmic reticulum (ER), the nuclear envelope reveals, besides the specific structures such as the pore complexes mentioned above, a number of specific biochemical features: So, for instance, it is tightly associated with parts of the nuclear genome DNA (e.g., Du Praw, 1965; Jackson et al., 1968; Beams and Mueller, 1970 Berezney et al., 1970; Comings and Okada, 1970a and b; Franke et al., 1970; Deumling and Franke, 1971; Franke, 1971; Mizuno et al., 1971; Ormerod and Lehmann, 1971; Zentgraf et al., 1971). It also contains a membrane-bound RNA in the sense of Moulé (1968; see further e.g. Pitot et al., 1969) in a non-ionic type of interaction (e.g. Franke et al., 1970; Zentgraf et al., 1971) which, at least in terms of

---

1 The manifold problems of adjusting viable cells to anti-freeze agents have recently been summarized in a careful study by Fineran (1970) using plant material.

kinetics, appears distinct from the RNA bound to the rough ER (e.g., Smith et al.. 1969). A significant amount of this "nuclear membrane RNA" seems to be associated with the membrane material constituting the nuclear pores (for recent discussions see, e.g., Mentre, 1969; Franke and Scheer, 1970a and b; Franke and Falk, 1970; Scheer, 1970 and 1971; Jarasch et al., 1971). In addition, the nuclear envelope shows various enzymatic differences to other cytomembranes and can even be distinguished from the ER, as has hitherto been established for diverse membrane-bound phosphohydrolases and redox activities, including the electron transfering pigments. This has been shown in particular with mammalian liver (Jarasch, 1969; Kashnig and Kasper, 1969; Kuzmina et al., 1969; Zbarsky et al., 1969; Berezney et al., 1970b; Franke et al., 1970; Kasper, 1971; Jarasch et al., 1971) and with the calf thymus (Ueda et al., 1969; Betel, 1970; Conover, 1970a and b; Reilly, 1971; Rupec and Sekeris, 1971). Peculiarities of the nuclear membrane enzymology have also been noted with the hen erythrocyte (Zentgraf et al., 1971). A certain distinctiveness of the nuclear membrane has also been noted at the membrane lipid level (e.g., Keenan et al., 1970; Kleinig, 1970; Kleinig et al., 1971; Stadler and Kleinig, 1971). On the background of the membrane differentiation hypothesis as outlined by Grove et al. (1968) in a sequence nuclear envelope→rough ER→smooth ER→Golgi apparatus→plasma membrane (see also Morre et al., 1971), the nuclear envelope should consequently be considered as being structurally and biochemically representing something like the "least differentiated" cytomembrane in a eukaryotic cell. Therefore, information on this particular type of endomembrane would be especially helpful in understanding common principles and diversities among the different classes of membranes in eukaryotic cell systems. With respect to the membrane structures, as revealed with the freeze-etch technique, an investigation of the nuclear envelope is all the more required, since its counterpart at the other end of the membrane differentiation sequence sketched above, namely the plasma membrane, is the type of membrane for which so far the vast majority of the today's freeze-etch information has been accumulated.

For this purpose, and in particular in order to examine the general architectural principles beyond the pecularities of one cell type, we chose the following widely divergent cellular systems: (a) Mature rat liver parenchyma, since this is a "reference" mammalian tissue cell which provides a good example of a differentiated steady-state cell system and in which a lot of work on the nuclear envelope structure, chemistry and function has already been done in many laboratories (see, e.g., Watson, 1959; Kashnig and Kasper, 1969; Zbarsky et al., 1969; Franke, 1970; Franke et al., 1970; Kleinig, 1970; Franke et al., 1971). (b) The hen erythrocyte as a cell system in an extreme "dead end differentiation" with an almost totally inactive nucleus. Moreover, with this object some chemical and structural details of the nuclear envelope are also known (compare, e.g., Davies, 1968; Zentgraf et al., 1969; Zentgraf et al., 1971). (c) The amphibian oocyte represents a special cell type with a giant nucleus which can be isolated manually, i.e. with a relatively gentle method. With this cell there is also a considerable background of knowledge on the structure, composition and function of the nuclear envelope (Gall, 1954, 1956, and 1967; Clerot, 1968; Scheer, 1970; e.g. Franke and Scheer, 1970a and b). (d) The marine haptophycean alga *Pleuro-*

chrysis scherffelii is a lower plant cell which is particularly suitable for freeze-etch studies, because neither a prestabilization nor an "anti-freeze agent" is necessary with this organism.

Materials and Methods

Rat liver tissue, hen erythrocytes, amphibian oocytes and axenic vegetative cultures of the yellow-green alga *Pleurochrysis scherffelii* were prepared according to the following procedures.

Rat Liver

Pieces of liver tissue from freshly decapitated albino rats (Wistar 2, 160–180 g) were fixed and prepared for thin section electron microscopy using the methods previously described (Franke *et al.*, 1969, 1970). For freeze-etching the tissue was prestabilized with 2% glutaraldehyde in 0.1 M sodium cacodylate buffer (pH 7.2) for 30 min, then glycerinated via a 15 min passage in 15% glycerol to a final concentration of 25% glycerol (the glycerol in a Ringer solution). After another 15 min the tissue was rapidly frozen in liquid Freon 22. The freeze-etching was performed using the method modified from Moor (Moor et al., 1961; Moor and Mühlethaler, 1963; Moor, 1964; Moor, 1969a) as described below.

The isolation of nuclei was carried out according to the method of Franke et al. (1970). Nuclear membranes were prepared by hypotonic shock and subsequent sonication as described by Franke (1966 and 1967) for mouse liver, i.e. without any high salt extraction, and were then negatively stained with 2% sodium phosphotungstate (pH 7.2).

Hen Erythrocytes

Freshly prepared blood from decapitated hens (Rhodeländer) was allowed to drop into Ringer solution which was 2% with respect to the anticoagulate Liquemin (Hoffmann La Roche AG, Grenzach, Baden, Germany) at 38° C and was gently centrifuged for 10 min at 100 g. After two washings with the same medium, the erythrocytes were suspended in 10% glycerol, followed by 25% for 20 min per each step. For freeze-etching the erythrocytes were frozen as described above.

Samples of erythrocytes were fixed and embedded for thin sectioning as previously described (Zentgraf et al., 1969, 1971). Negative staining preparations of isolated hen erythrocyte nuclear membranes were obtained as outlined in the same articles.

Amphibian Oocytes

Lampbrush oocytes (diameter 520 μm) of *Xenopus laevis Daudin* were collected from anesthesized animals and immediately immersed through 5 steps from 5% to 25% glycerol in amphibia Ringer with each step lasting 45 min or were fixed with 1% formaldehyde, buffered to pH 7.2 with cacodylate, prior to the glycerol incubation. The same oocyte stages were prepared for thin sectioning following the procedure described by Franke and Scheer (1970a).

Nuclei from *Xenopus laevis* lampbrush stage oocytes and mature *Triturus alpestris Laur.* oocytes were isolated (Franke and Scheer, 1970a) and fixed with Na-cacodylate buffered (0.1 M, pH 7.2) 2% glutaraldehyde in the cold, washed with "5:1 medium" (Callan and Lloyd, 1960) and incubated in 10%, 15% and 25% glycerol, respectively for 15 min per each concentration. (The glycerol was dissolved in "5:1 medium").

The isolated nuclei were also processed for thin sectioning and for negative staining preparations of the nuclear envelope as described in an earlier paper (Franke and Scheer, 1970a).

Pleurochrysis Scherffelii

The freeze-etching of this haptophycean (Chrysophyta) alga was carried out as described earlier (Brown et al., 1970; Brown and Franke, 1971). It should be emphasized that with this small organism no prefixation and glycerol incubation was needed. The organisms were directly frozen.

The liquid Freon 22 frozen specimens were stored in liquid nitrogen. Freeze-etching operations were carried out with a Balzer apparatus BA 360 M (Balzers AG, Liechtenstein) applying 90 sec etching at — 100° C.

Electron micrographs were made with a Siemens elmiscope 1 A. The magnification of the instrument was routinely controlled with a grating replica (the error was below 5%).

Calculations of the pore frequency in thin sectioning were made using a combination of the methods of Barnes and Davies (1959) and Sitte (1964).

The thicknesses of thin sections were calculated from interferometric data (for critical discussion of the methodical problems compare, e.g., Silvermann et al., 1969; Helander 1969; Sjöstrand, 1967).

Results and Discussion

The freeze-etching preparations produced cross as well as flat fractures of nuclei (e.g., Figs. 1–3). The direction of shadowing was routinely determined, usually from the orientation of the shadows at the plasma membrane "particles" (see below). Frequently, nuclear membrane faces were obtained representing up to half of the total nuclear surface area (e.g., Figs. 1 and 2). The aforementioned different cell systems revealed, beside some differences, a far reaching correspondence in nuclear envelope substructures.

1. Cross Fractures Through the Perinuclear Cisterna

Cross fractures through the nuclear envelope of the investigated animal and plant cells had an unswollen or only moderately swollen perinuclear cisterna bounded by the inner or the outer nuclear membrane which both occasionally revealed a dark-light-dark "unit membrane" appearance (Fig. 6). This unit membrane aspect in cross fracture, which has been shown also by other authors for different types of membranes (e.g. Moor and Mühlethaler, 1963; Branton and Moor, 1964; Branton, 1966; Bischoff and Moor, 1967; Bauer, 1968; Leak, 1968; Staehelin, 1968a; Branton, 1969, Meyer and Winkelmann, 1969; Nickel and Grieshaber, 1969; Fineran, 1970a; Keyhani, 1970; Spycher, 1970) is somewhat perplexing and is hard to explain on the basis of the current concepts on electron contrast formation after the freeze-etch shadowing procedures. Fuzzy, somewhat filamentous substructures are sometimes seen in the lumen of the perinuclear cisterna (e.g. Fig. 5; compare also Koehler, 1968a), but will not be interpreted in the view of the relatively low resolution power of the freeze-etch technique. The nuclear pores are recognized (Figs. 3, 5), with the inner and outer cisternal membrane somewhat converging at the sites where they fuse to constitute the pore walls. The substructural components of the nuclear pore complexes did not show up in the cross fractures (Figs. 3, 5). This is not surprising, since nucleoprotein-containing material is generally poorly profiled in freeze-etch preparations: usually ribosomal, chromosomal and nucleolar material is not or barely demonstrated with this technique. Only in certain cases, the nucleolus and the metaphase chromosomes appear somewhat prominent by a finer texture (e.g. Bullivant and Ames, 1966; Northcote and Lewis, 1968; Leak, 1970; Ryser, 1970). In this connection it is interesting to note that the annulus-associated fibrillar bundles characteristic for amphibian oocytes in thin section electron microscopy (Franke and Scheer, 1970a and b) can also be identified in cross fractures through isolated nuclei (Fig. 7).

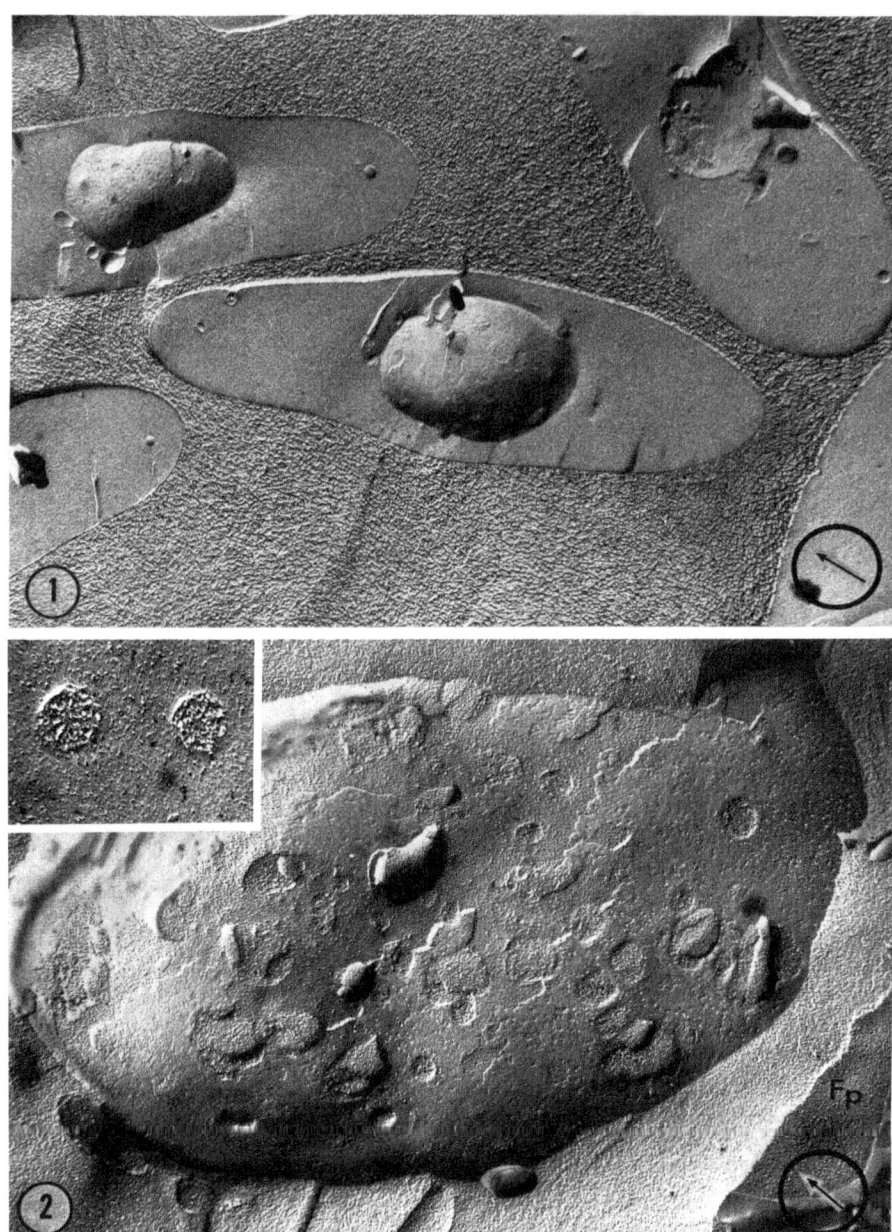

Figs. 1 and 2. Hen erythrocytes after freeze-cleaving. Fig. 1, gives a survey which demonstrates that this cell does not contain any considerable membranes beside the nuclear envelope. The two nuclei in the left are convex whereas the nucleus in the upper right is concavely fractured. Details of fracture faces are presented in the convexly broken nucleus of Fig. 2. Two faces are dominant (F'_o and F_i) from which the one (F_i) is set with particles, thus resembling the F plane of the plasma membrane (F_p). Holes in the fractured nuclear envelope, which at least partially represent nuclear pores or spatially correspond to nuclear pores, are recognized. These pores (insert) do not reveal distinct substructures but appear to be "filled" with a coarsely textured ground-substance. Fig. 1, 12000:1; Fig. 2, 46000:1; Insert of Fig. 2, 56000:1

Encircled arrows in all illustrations of this article indicate the direction of shadowing

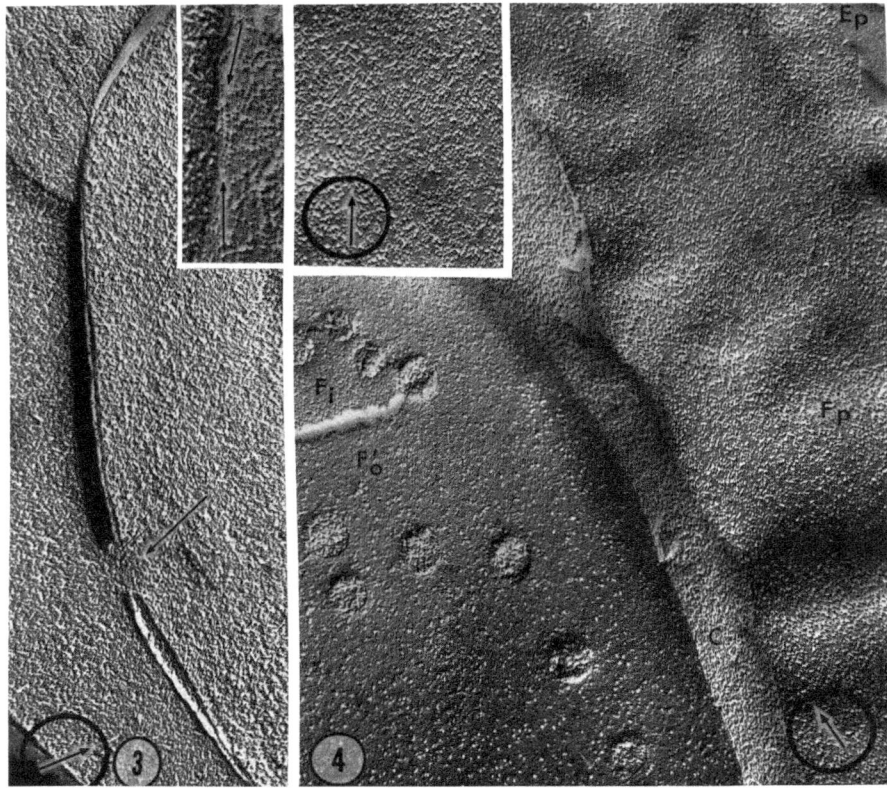

Fig. 3. Cross-fracture through a hen erythrocyte nuclear envelope. No substructural details are recognized at the nuclear pores (arrow). The nucleoplasm appears homogeneously textured. No differences in texture are apparent between nucleo- and cytoplasm. Only infrequently, regular arrangements are suggested within the peripheral chromatin (insert) Magnification, 38000:1; insert 72000:1

Fig. 4. Membrane fracture faces of the hen erythrocyte. The plasma membrane surface (E_p in the upper right), which is set only by a few very small particles, lies on top of the particle-rich F-plane (F_p). The insert shows the relatively homogeneous distribution of such ca. 85 Å particles on the F_p face. With the nuclear envelope one recognizes a particle-bearing face (F_i) lying underneath a fracture plane with less particles and occasional holes (F'_0). C cytoplasm. Magnification, 34000:1; insert 45000:1

In many cells the nucleoplasmic surface of the nuclear envelope is underlined by a highly condensed heterochromatin (Davies, 1968; Everid et al., 1970; compare the reviews of Kaye, 1969, and Stevens and Andre, 1969). In mature nucleated erythrocytes Davies (1968) has described this chromatin immediately underneath the nuclear membrane to be arranged in distinct and ordered 130–170 Å tubular aggregates. From the mere point of dimensions, structures of this size should be easily resolved with the shadowing technique (see Moor, 1969a). With mammalian sperm nuclei Koehler (1966, 1970) described ordered substructures within the condensed sperm deoxyribonucleo-proteins. Although

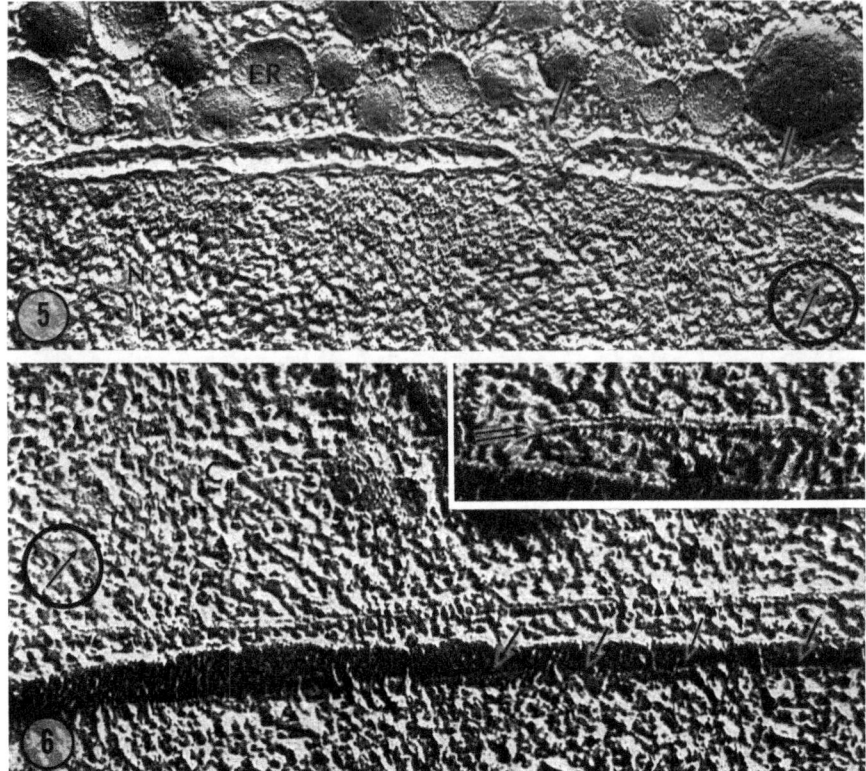

Figs. 5 and 6. Cross-fractures through the nuclear envelope of a rat liver parenchymal cell. Nuclear pore complexes do not show structural details (arrows in Fig. 5). The nuclear membranes can reveal a dark-light-dark triple-layer pattern resembling the "unit-membrane"-appearance of thin section electron microscopy (Fig. 6, insert). Within the perinuclear cisterna sometimes fibrillar fuzzes are visualized (Fig. 5). The arrows in Fig. 6 denote a transition line from the nucleoplasmic surface of the inner membrane (E_{in}) to the fracture plane of the same membrane (F'_i). Fig. 5, 62000:1; Fig. 6, 65000; insert of Fig. 6, 84000:1

we could confirm the structures described by Davies (1968) with the mature hen erythrocytes in thin sections (c.f. Zentgraf, 1969) such nucleoplasmic sub-architecture, however, was not clearly identifiable after the freeze-etch procedure. The only structure which could be discerned in a close association with the inner aspect of the nuclear envelope is a certain striation pattern with a repetitive lateral distance of 210–320 Å and more or less regularly spaced chains of 100–180 Å large globules (e.g., Fig. 3). Related structures were recognized in freeze-etch micrographs of other authors (e.g. Koehler, 1968b; Leak, 1968; Kouri et al., 1970). The question as to whether these inner nuclear membrane-associated heterochromatin strands described from the conventional thin electron microscopy are "artifacts" of the dehydration steps or whether they cannot be demonstrated with the freeze-etch technique as such is under investigation.

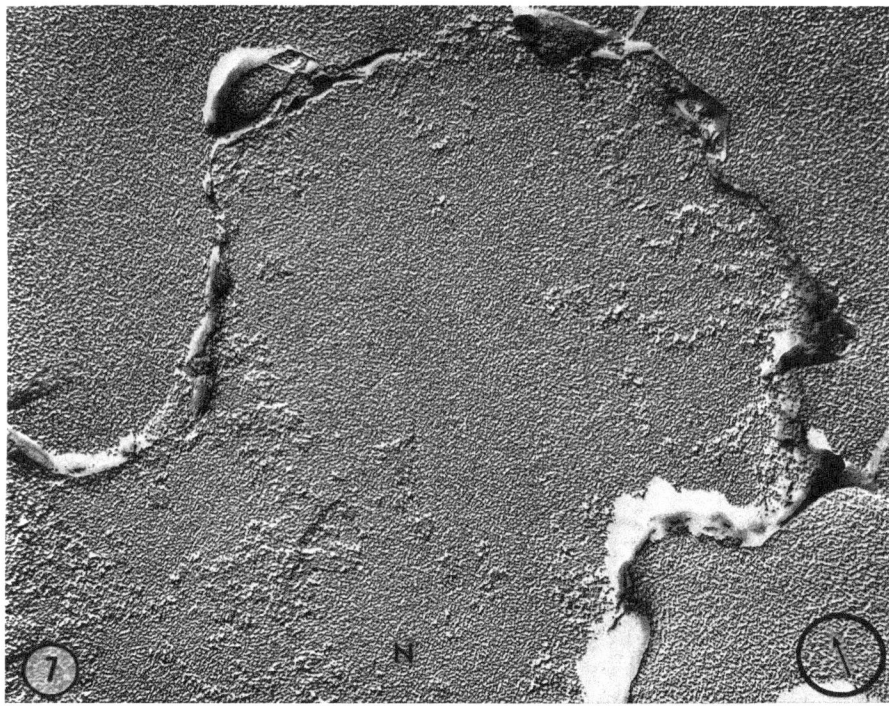

Fig. 7. Cross-fracture through the nuclear envelope of a mature oocyte nucleus isolated from *Triturus alpestris* (stabilized with glutaraldehyde followed by glycerol, treatment). In the nucleoplasm (*N*) the strands of fibrillar material, which are known from thin section electron microscopy to terminate at the inner annulus of the pore complexes, can be identified by its coarser texture. Magnification 36 000:1

Although the interest of most freeze-etch studies is strongly focused upon the appearances of membranes, it is worth mentioning that principally the freeze-etch technique is able to sculpture non-membranous structures too; may they be proteins or nucleoproteins, either lying free in the nucleoplasm, in the cytoplasm or in the matrix of organelles. So for instance, cytoplasmic and nucleoplasmic microtubules have been demonstrated with the use of this technique (e.g., Moor, 1967; Brown and Franke, 1971) both in cross and in longitudinal splintering, whereas such has yet been unsuccessful with the ciliary microtubules (Satir and Gilula, 1970). Moreover, Brown and Franke (1971) were able to show the about 50 Å broad cross-bridges between microtubules in the frozen-etched Pleurochrysis cells. In addition to the above quoted demonstration of nucleoli and chromosomes in freeze-cleaving preparations (for the almost non-protein-complexed deoxyribonucleic acid of dinophycean chromosomes, see also Giesbrecht, 1965), Easterbrook and Rozee (1971) recently provided another example of the demonstration of nucleoprotein structures with the freeze-etch technique in their micrographs of the cytoplasmic virions in rheovirus-infected rhesus monkey kidney cells. Various freeze-etch investigations were concerned with the structure of actomyosin in diverse sorts of musculature (e.g., Rayns et al., 1968a and b; Bertaud et al., 1970) and with the microfilaments of epithelial cells (e. g., Mukerjhee and Staehelin, 1971) which are purely proteinaceous non-membrane structures. Even the typical lattice-spacing of special protein-containing paracrystalline aggregates like, e. g., of the yolk in the platelets of the amphibian oocytes (Zentgraf and Scheer, 1971) and in the gas vacuole "membranes" (e.g., Jost and Jones, 1970) was identifiable in frozen-cleaved preparations. An example of a non-membranous structure within a bacterial cell that could be shown with the freeze-etch technique is the polar organell of Rhodopseudomonas palustris (Tauschel and Speth, 1970).

2. Fracture Planes and Membrane Surfaces

As in other membranes the freeze-etched membranes of the nuclear envelope revealed different surfaces and fracture planes. Although the discussion on the question where the fracture planes run along is still going on, the evidence currently accumulating favors the concept originally introduced by Branton (1966a), which states that the splintering occurs within the membrane and thus exposes "inner surfaces" for the subsequent shadowing procedure (Branton, 1966, 1967; Branton and Park, 1967; Clark and Branton, 1968; Engström and Branton, 1968; Branton, 1969; Meyer and Winkelmann, 1969; Park and Pfeifhofer, 1969a and b; Chalcroft and Bullivant, 1970; Fineran, 1970a; Meyer and Winkelmann, 1970; McNutt and Weinstein, 1970; da Silva and Branton, 1970; Spycher, 1970; Watson and Remsen, 1970; Tillack and Marchesi, 1970; Weinstein et al., 1970; Buttrose, 1971).[2] A different view is the freeze-fracture interpretation of Moor and Mühlethaler (1963), namely that the splintering reveals two "in vivo" membrane surfaces (for this view of membrane splintering see e.g., Remsen and Lundgren, 1966; Remsen et al., 1967; Weinstein and Bullivant, 1967; Bauer, 1968; Remsen, 1968; Staehelin, 1968b; Weinstein and Koo, 1968; Friederici, 1969; Moor, 1969a; Nickel and Grieshaber, 1969; Wallach, 1969; Bajer and Remsen, 1970; Nanninga, 1970), or the modification therefrom by Staehelin (1968a) who advocated "fracture planes running at different levels through or along the upperlying halves of the membranes" (e.g. also Staehelin et al., 1969; van Gool et al., 1970; Sleytr, 1970; Staehelin and Kiermayer, 1970; Plattner et al., 1969).

The nuclear envelope with its two cisternal membranes on a more or less curved surface provides, due to the advantage of orientation, a useful system for examining the current hypothesis on membrane surface fracturing. The interpretations given in the majority of the previous freeze-etch studies dealing with aspects of nuclear membranes were controversial to the concept of Branton (1966a) and tended to follow the view that true membrane surfaces, either plasmatic or intracisternal, are seen after the freeze-etch procedures (e.g. Moor and Mühlethaler, 1963; Branton and Moor, 1964; Koehler, 1968b; Northcote and Lewis, 1968; Leak, 1968; Allen and Hess, 1969; Moor, 1969b; Bertaud et al., 1970; Bererhi and Malkani, 1970; Speth and Wunderlich, 1970; Holt and Stern, 1970; Keyhani, 1970; Wecke and Giesbrecht, 1970). Our results are basi-

---

[2] For other special controversial cases of membrane fracturing compare also the articles by Branton and Southworth (1967) and Ruska and Ruska (1969).

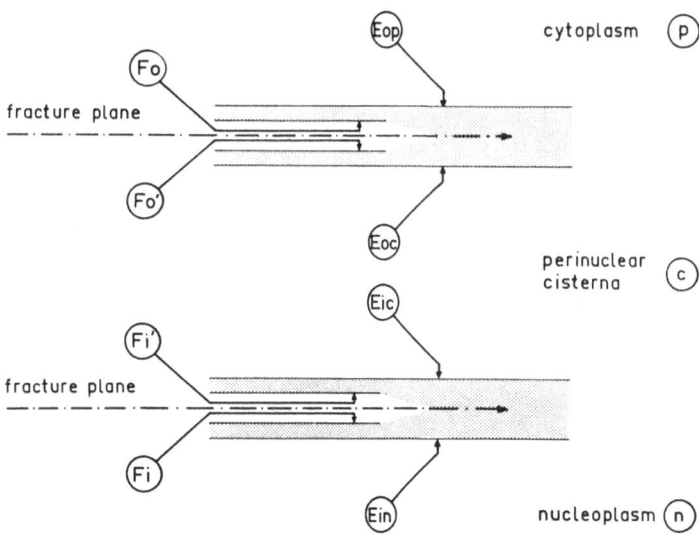

Fig. 8. Interpretative diagram of the nuclear envelope faces exposed after the freeze-etch process including "true membrane surfaces" as well as those exposed by the fracturing (fracture plane ≙ inner membrane faces"). Symbols: E_{op} "Etched surface of the cytoplasmic side of the outer membrane. E_{oc} "Etched surface of the cisternal side of the outer membrane. E_{ic} "Etched" surface of the cisternal side of the inner membrane. E_{in} "Etched" surface of the nucleoplasmic side of the inner membrane. F_o and F'_o the two corresponding fracture faces of the outer membrane. F_i and F'_i the two corresponding fracture faces of the inner membrane

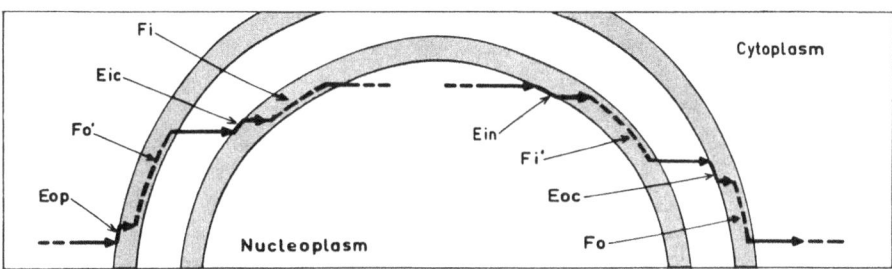

Fig. 9. Schematic illustration of a typical fracturing through the nuclear envelope, combining both directions, C (ytoplasm) → N (ucleoplasm) and vice versa, →NC. E-faces appear limited to relatively small areas along the F-faces

cally in agreement with Branton's concept and shall be presented in the following using the explanative nomenclature given in Fig. 8. With all the cell types studied, the freeze-etch procedure consistently revealed a total of 8 different membrane faces of the nuclear envelope (compare the schemes in Figs. 8 and 9). Among them, three different aspects can be distinguished.

I. One face is characteristically set with particles of a diameter of 60—130 Å in a relatively dense package (e.g. Figs. 4, 12—22, 24, 32). This cobble-stoned pattern strongly resembles the corresponding aspect of the plasma membrane (e.g. Figs. 2, 4 and 16) as has been demonstrated by various authors for mammalian erythrocytes (e.g. Weinstein and Bullivant, 1967; Koehler, 1968 b; Weinstein and Koo, 1968; Meyer and Winkelmann, 1969; Nickel and Grieshaber, 1969; Wallach, 1969; DaSilva and Branton, 1970; Meyer and Winkelmann, 1970; Tillack and Marchesi, 1970; Tillack et al., 1970 a) and also from plasma membranes of other cell types (e.g. Moor and Mühlethaler, 1963; Remsen et al., 1967; Northcote, 1968; Remsen, 1968; Staehelin, 1968 b; Fill and Branton, 1969; Chalcroft and Bullivant, 1970; Nanninga, 1970; Spycher, 1970). From the detailed work of Tillack and Marchesi (1970) and DaSilva and Branton (1970; see also DaSilva et al., 1970) it is established that these particles are true elevations above the fracture face level and not indentations. It might be interesting to note in this connection that with the hen erythrocyte plasma membrane the present authors could routinely observe the two faces described by DaSilva and Branton (1970) and Tillack and Marchesi (1970), namely the fracture face set with particles and, usually ca. 30–45 Å on top of that, the more smoothly appearing "etched surface" (e.g. Fig. 4).

II. Another membrane aspect is characterized by the existence of much fewer particles (60–130 Å in diameter) which can be accompanied by relatively distinct small holes in the order of 60–150 Å.

III. A third membrane aspect was observed in very small areas limited to the margins along the splintering steps. As a consequence of this size limitation, a decision whether it is set by particles or is smooth was hardly possible (e.g. Figs. 10, 11, 13–19). However, in a few examples one could recognize some particles on this face, too (e.g. Figs. 10 and 11).

From the splintering cascade through the nuclear envelope in nucleo-cytoplasmic direction or vice versa, it was possible to arrange all the membrane aspects obtained into an interpretative sequence (Figs. 8 and 9). Such an interpretation was somewhat facilitated by the fact that concave as well as convex nuclear replicas were found side by side and thus did allow an orientation (e.g. Fig. 1): Two surfaces interpreted as being the "etched" true surfaces of the outer nuclear membrane toward the cytoplasm (E_{op}) and of the inner nuclear membrane toward the nucleoplasm (E_{in}), are exposed only in very limited areas with a fracture rim (e.g. Fig. 11) and belong to the membrane aspect described above under III. The maximum width of this rim ever found in the course of this study was 350 Å. A step which could be calculated from the direction and the angle of shadowing (see Müller, 1942) as having a depth of roughly 35 Å leads from this membrane surface plane down to a plane with a typical No. II aspect. Therefore, this latter plane must represent the interior of the specific membrane which has been exposed by the fracturing, since the total thickness of either nuclear membrane is 110 ± 20 Å as determined from cross-fractures. Depending on the direction of fracturing this membrane aspect, which can occupy relatively large areas, represents either the fracture face called F'_i with the inner or F'_o with the outer nuclear membrane. Frequently, the superficial part of the specific membrane, i.e. the membrane moiety which lies between the E_{op} or E_{in} surfaces, respectively and the following F-plane appears to be extremely reduced and almost cross-fractured so that the first face exposed in these cases is the specific F-plane (e.g., Figs. 12–14): The chisel apparently tends

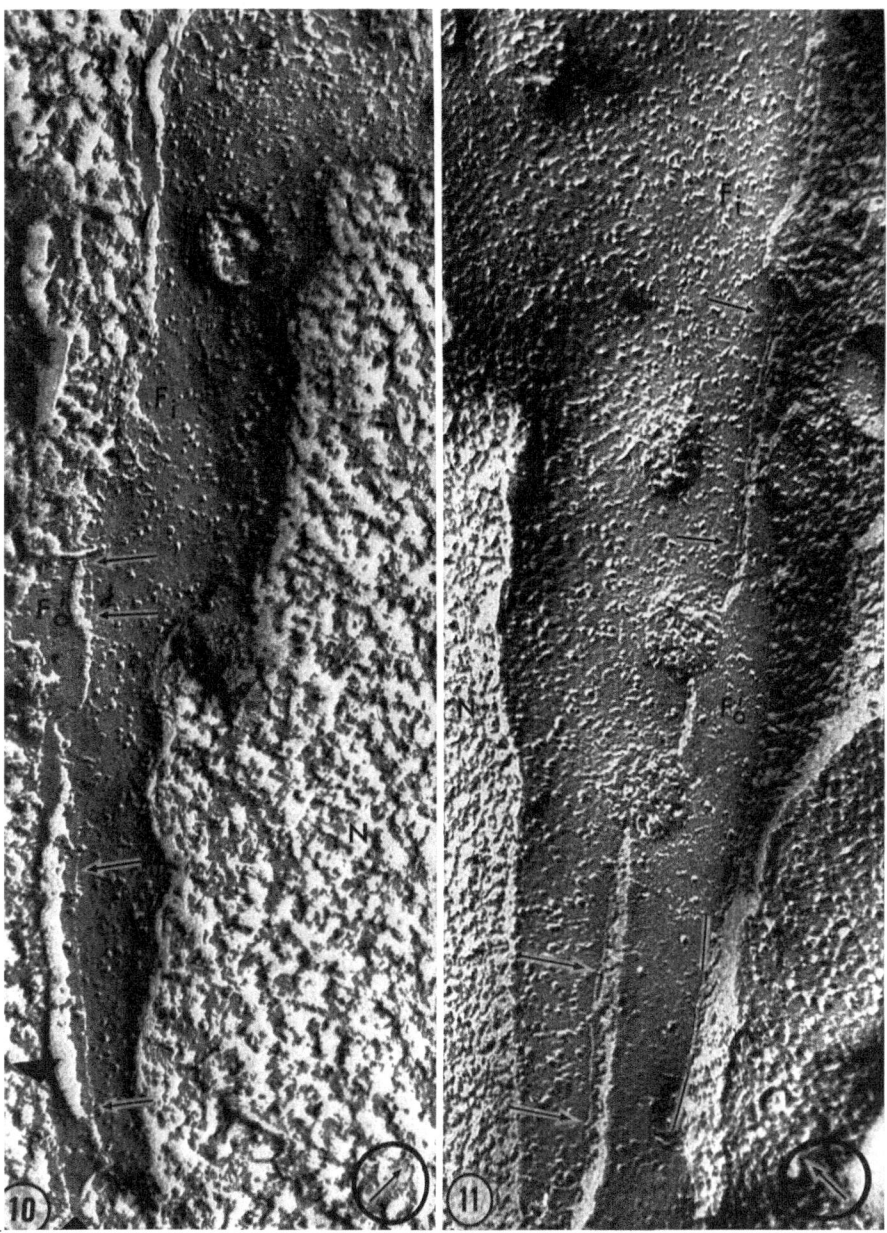

Figs. 10 and 11. Details of fracture face transitions in the frozen nuclear envelope of a rat hepatocyte. A transition from a cytoplasmic surface plane (E_{oc}) to the about 40 Å deeper F'_o fracture plane is indicated between the black triangles in the lower part of Fig. 10 and between the bars of Fig. 11. Thence a much deeper step follows which corresponds to the perinuclear space plus approximately half a membrane width. The next plane recognized is the cisternal surface of the inner nuclear membrane (E_{ic}) which can be identified as a small rim along the trans-cisternal fracture line (e.g. between the arrows). This layer lies about 40 Å on top of the F_i fracture plane, which is characterized by its distinct particles.

Fig. 10, 125000:1; Fig. 11, 105000:1

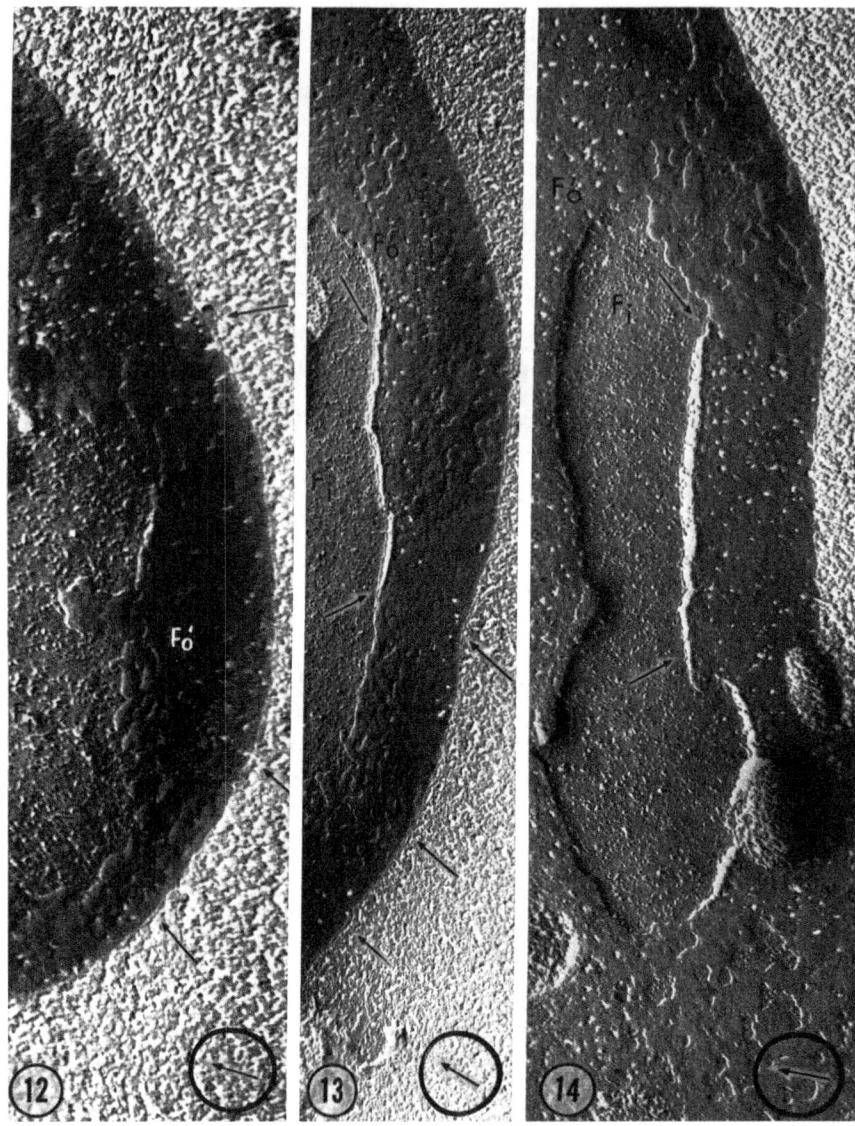

Figs. 12–14. Details of the transitions between membrane faces in frozen-cleaved nuclear envelopes in hen erythrocytes. The arrows in Fig. 12 denote a 35–50 Å deep step from the surface (E_{op}) to the F'_o plane. In addition to that, Figs. 13 and 14 show parts of a membranous face which is recognized along the $F'_o \rightarrow F_i$ transition rims and which (between the arrows of Fig. 14 and the upper arrows of Fig. 13) lies about 30–50 Å on top of the F_i fracture. This face is interpreted as being the cisternal surface of the inner nuclear membrane (E_{ic}), which favourably appears after long "etching times". Note that some parts of the F'_o face appear totally "smooth", e.g. in the upper and lower right of Fig. 11. Fig. 12, 95000:1; Fig. 13, 65000:1; Fig. 14, 66000:1

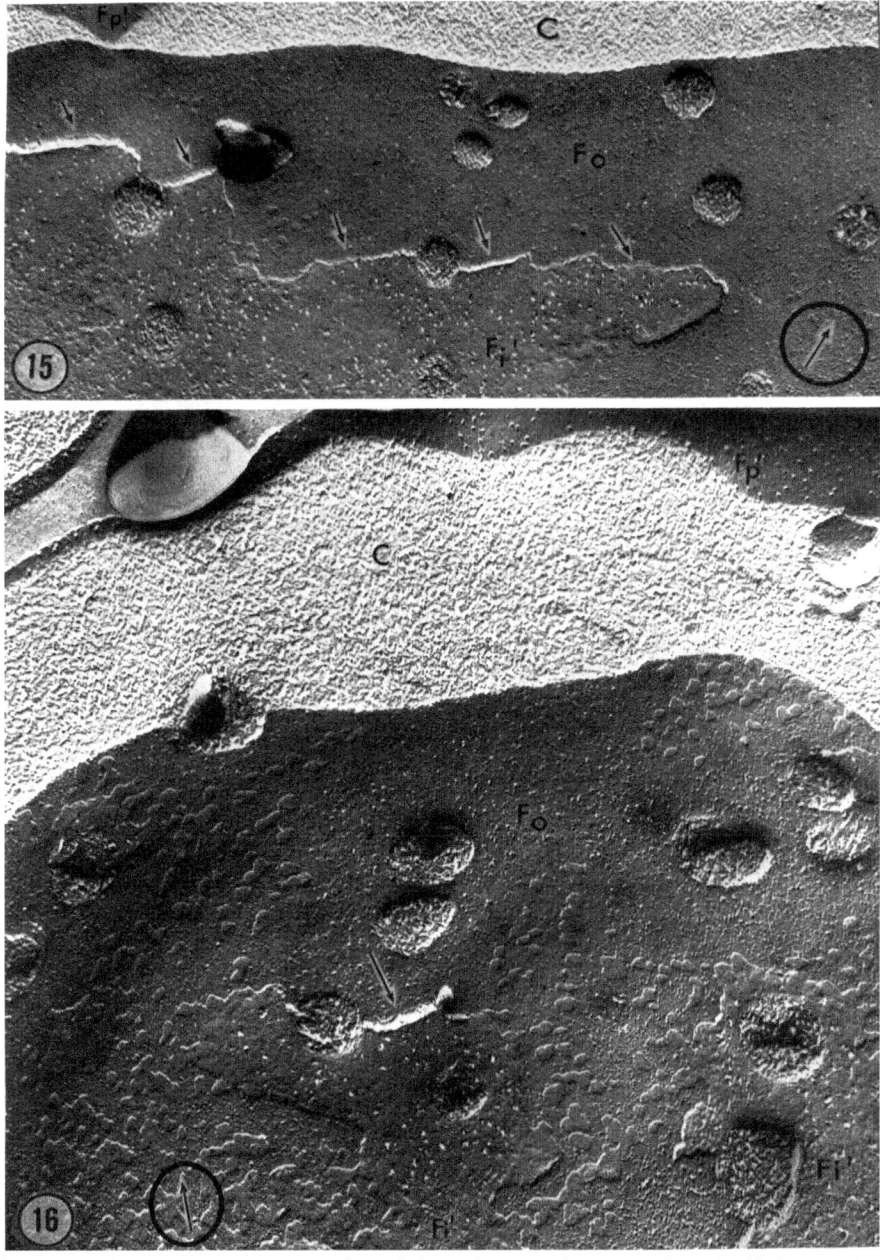

Figs. 15 and 16. Concave fractures through frozen hen erythrocytes. Here the F'_i face of the inner nuclear membrane lies on top of a small rim of E_{oc} (arrows) separated by a relatively deep interspace (e.g. at the arrow in Fig. 16), which corresponds to the width of the perinuclear cisterna. Then after another step of 30–50 Å one has arrived at the fracture plane F_o in the outer nuclear membrane. Then the cytoplasm comes, followed by a membranous fracture face of the plasma membrane (F'_p) which is different from the afore described F_p face by having less particles. With the nuclear envelope note the holes which vary in diameter and may correspond to nuclear pores. Fig. 15, 41 000:1; Fig. 16, 60 000:1

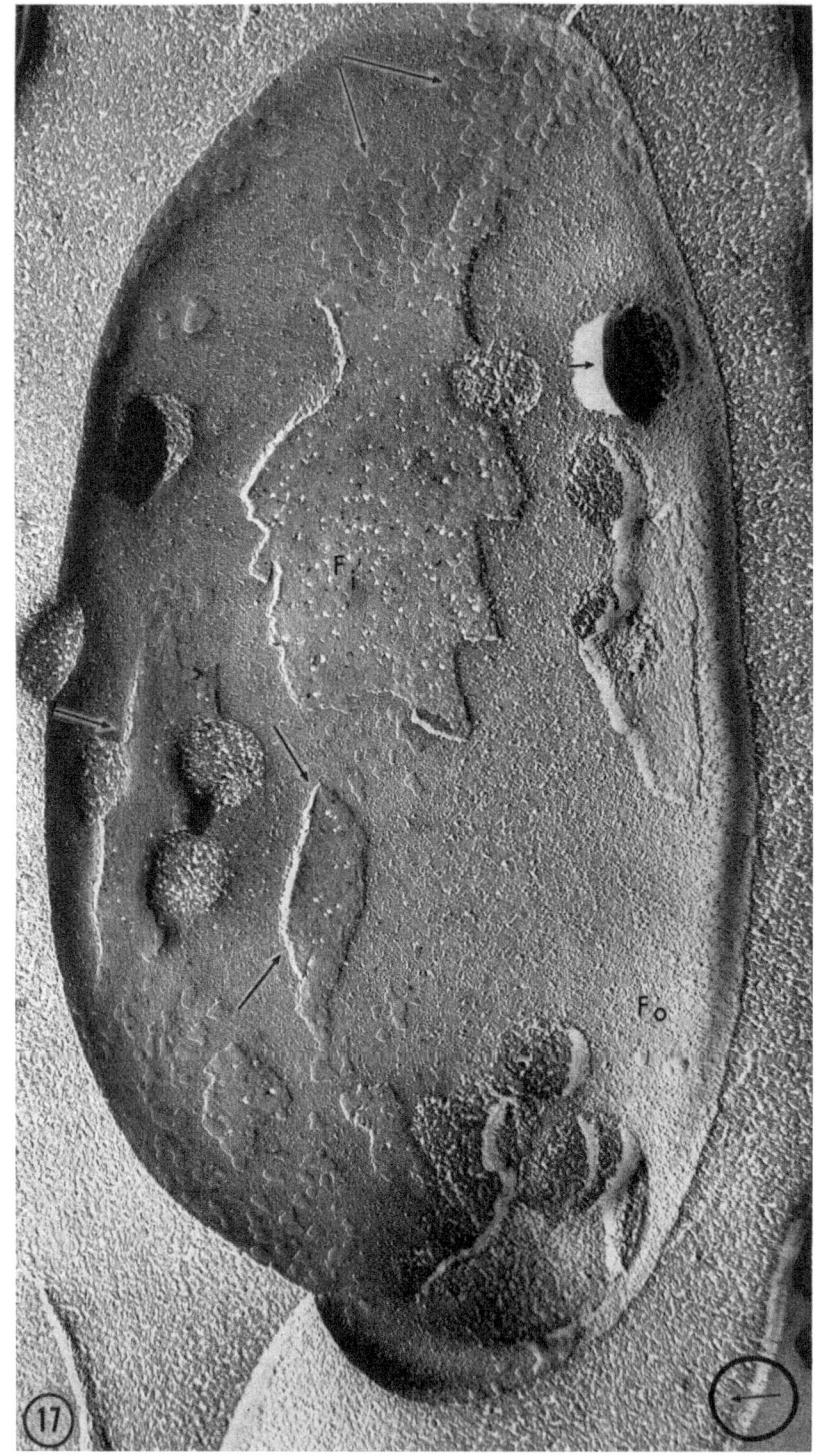

Fig. 17

to cut through the "coat parts" of the membranes and follows the F-planes. The step following in fracturing is very steep with a range from 130–500 $Å^3$ and runs through the perinuclear cisterna by either going directly (e.g., Figs. 12, 22, 23) to a fracture surface with a No. I aspect, i.e. densely set with the characteristic particles, or to a face of the No. III type as an intermediate (e.g. Figs. 10, 11, 13–17, 18, 19). This latter surface again tends to occupy only small areas along the fissure rims and lies about 35 Å on top of the particle-rich fracture face. The only possible interpretation is, in the authors' opinion, that the No. III aspect rim areas represent the intracisternal surface of either the outer or the inner membrane, depending on the specific direction of fracturing. So they correspond to the planes E_{ic} or E_{oc} of the schemes presented in Figs. 8 and 9. Following the concepts of DaSilva and Branton (1970) and Tillack and Marchesi (1970) it might be possible that a certain depth of etching is required to expose such surfaces to the shadowing process. Consequently, the No. I membrane aspect, which usually covers large areas, is another inner fracture face, namely either the plane F_i or F_o respectively, depending on the fracture direction. From comparing the concave and convex nuclear fractures (compare, e.g., Fig. 2 with Fig. 17), it was possible to determine that the two fracture faces, namely the membrane aspect No. I and No. II corresponding to the inner membrane fracture faces occur in either nuclear membrane and that the nuclear membranes with respect to their fracture planes obey a mirror image symmetry with its specular plane in the middle of the perinuclear cisterna and being coincident with the equatorial plane of the nuclear pore complexes.

In either sequence the breakage can finally leave the specific membrane and splinter through the nucleoplasm (e.g., Fig. 10), if one fracture from the cytoplasm (i.e. the breakage line leaves the plane F_i) or through the cytoplasm, if it comes from the nucleoplasm (i.e. the fracture line leaves the plane F_o). Often the fracture gives rise to the appearance of small islets of a "prime" plane (F'_i or F'_o) on a "non-prime" plane (e.g., Figs. 16, 17, 22, 28). The distance between such a "prime" fracture plane to a "non-prime" plane necessarily reflects the width of the perinuclear space, since it includes two "half-membranes" plus the cisterna. It is particularly interesting to note that such breakage lines, which lead from a "prime" fracture plane to a "non-prime" fracture plane (or vice versa), are marked by fracture holes representing (or at least corresponding to) pore

---

[3] The relatively wide range of the "height differences" from an inner fracture face of one cisternal membrane to the other might be explained by either in vivo differences in the cisternal width of the nuclear envelope or by different degrees in artificial swelling during the fixation and/or glycerol treatments.

Fig. 17. Hen erythrocyte nucleus in concave fracture. Again the particle-rich fracture face (in this case F_o) is covered by a "prime" face with less particles and occasional holes (F'_i). At the transitions between both (arrows in the lower left) a small rim of another face is seen, presumably the cisternal surface of the outer nuclear membrane. Often one visualizes small islets of the "prime" face on the F_o plane which appears smooth (upper arrows). Note that the material presumed to correspond to a nuclear pore complex appears as protruding stump (arrow-head in the right). Magnification, 54 000:1

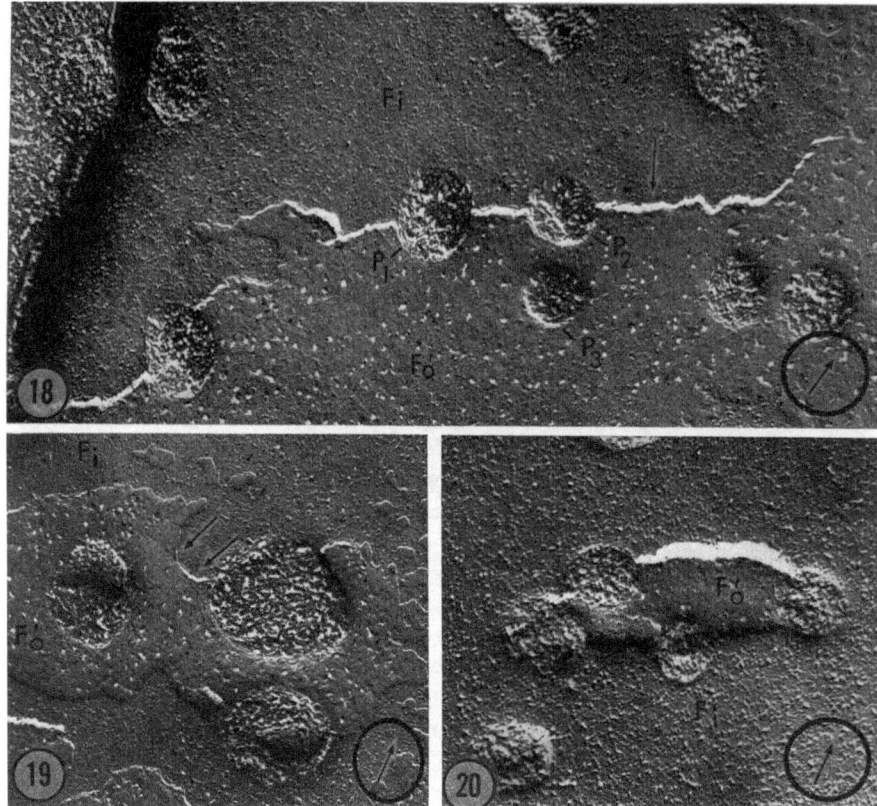

Figs. 18–20. Details of the appearance of the "nuclear pore-corresponding holes" in fractured nuclear envelope of the hen erythrocyte. The appearance of the pores does not show differences according to their association with a "prime" or "non-prime" fracture face (e.g. Fig. 19). Often such pores or "pore-corresponding fracture holes" seem to demarcate the lines of transition of one F plane to the other (e.g. Fig. 18). The islets of membrane material with a "prime" fracture face lying upon particle-rich "non-prime" faces are suggested to be preferentially maintained around the nuclear pore complexes (Figs. 19 and 20). E_{ic} rims are indicated by the arrows. Fig. 18, 61 000:1; Fig. 19, 56 000:1; Fig. 20, 63 000:1

complexes (e.g., Figs. 11, 18–20, 23, 25, 37). This can also be seen from a micrograph published by Hess (1968; Fig. 12 of this article) and supports the general impression that the nuclear pore complexes are places at which a change in fracturing from one membrane to the other is somewhat facilitated.

An especially frequent result of the nuclear envelope splintering process is that small or bizarre shaped plaques of a membrane with a No. II or III aspect stood upon the particle-rich membrane aspect No. I. For such very small plaques a clear distinction whether they represent a "prime" plane or an intracisternal surface (E_{oc} or E_{ic}) is not possible. Although the face of such plaques sometimes seems to be in continuity with a typical "prime" face (e.g., Figs. 16 and 19) one might, on the other hand, interpret them as showing "E" type true surfaces as is particularly suggested from the observation of similar plaques on, e.g., the frozen-fractured plant cell tonoplast which is a single membrane (e.g. Fig. 14 of Fineran, 1970b).

It is a significant result of this freeze-etch examination of the nuclear envelope that plasmatic (nucleo- and cytoplasmic) and cisternal surfaces are exposed by the freeze-etch procedure only in very limited areas along the fracture rims and that the surfaces exposed predominantly are inner surfaces according to the splintering scheme of Branton (1966). We tend to assume, that the nuclear membrane surfaces shown in the micrographs of previous authors, which have been interpreted as demonstrating "true" membrane surfaces with a structural surface specificity, in fact represent inner membrane fracture planes. Differences between inner and outer nuclear membrane with respect to the specific appearance of these fracture planes were not observed in the cell system examined in the present investigation.

There are many other cytological situations which resemble the perinuclear cisternae in the respect that two membranes are parallel in a relatively constant distance below ca. 500 Å: such are, e.g., the myelin sheath, the gap and the septate junctions, the tight junctions, the stacks of thylakoidal membranes and the dictyosomal stacks. In such situations one might expect, on the basis of the interpretative fracture concept shown in Fig. 2, that wherever a fracture step occurs from one membrane to an adjacent one rims were to observe which represent an E surface plane ("true membrane surface"). Surprisingly, this could not be documented with the myocardium nexuses ("D-plane of McNutt and Weinstein, 1971) even though these authors carefully looked for it. They can be recognized, however, in the micrographs of the frozen-etched septate junctions of the mussell gill epithelium (Gilula et al., 1970) and have also been demonstrated with the nerve myelin membranes by Branton (1967) and the thylakoidal associations (e.g., Park and Pfeifhofer, 1969a; Arntzen et al., 1969). Moreover such rims have also been observed in the rat liver Golgi apparatus (Zentgraf et al., 1971). Far from being able to explain this diversity in fracture behaviour among different membrane associations, we would like to discuss in interpreting freeze-etch aspects the general possibility that different types of membranes might show differences in response to the freeze-cleaving procedure. Since experimental membranology accumulates evidences of diversities in membrane composition and architecture among different types of membranes (for recent reviews see, e.g., O'Brien, 1967; Sjöstrand, 1963 and 1968; Morré et al., 1968 and 1969; Sitte, 1969) it appears to be oversimplified to discuss the freeze-cleaving of "membranes" in an a priori generalized way. For instance, the differences in the specific qualitative and quantitative lipid compositions of diverse types of membranes, which are thought to influence the stability and the specific molecular association, should also somehow influence their freeze-cleaving behaviour, according to the essence of Branton's idea that the fracture tends to run in the plane of maximal hydrophobic interaction (Branton, 1966, 1967).

The mere fact that the membrane-associated particles of this order of magnitude can be found in quite different cell types with quite different types of membranes suggests that their validity as membrane-markers in freeze-etch studies

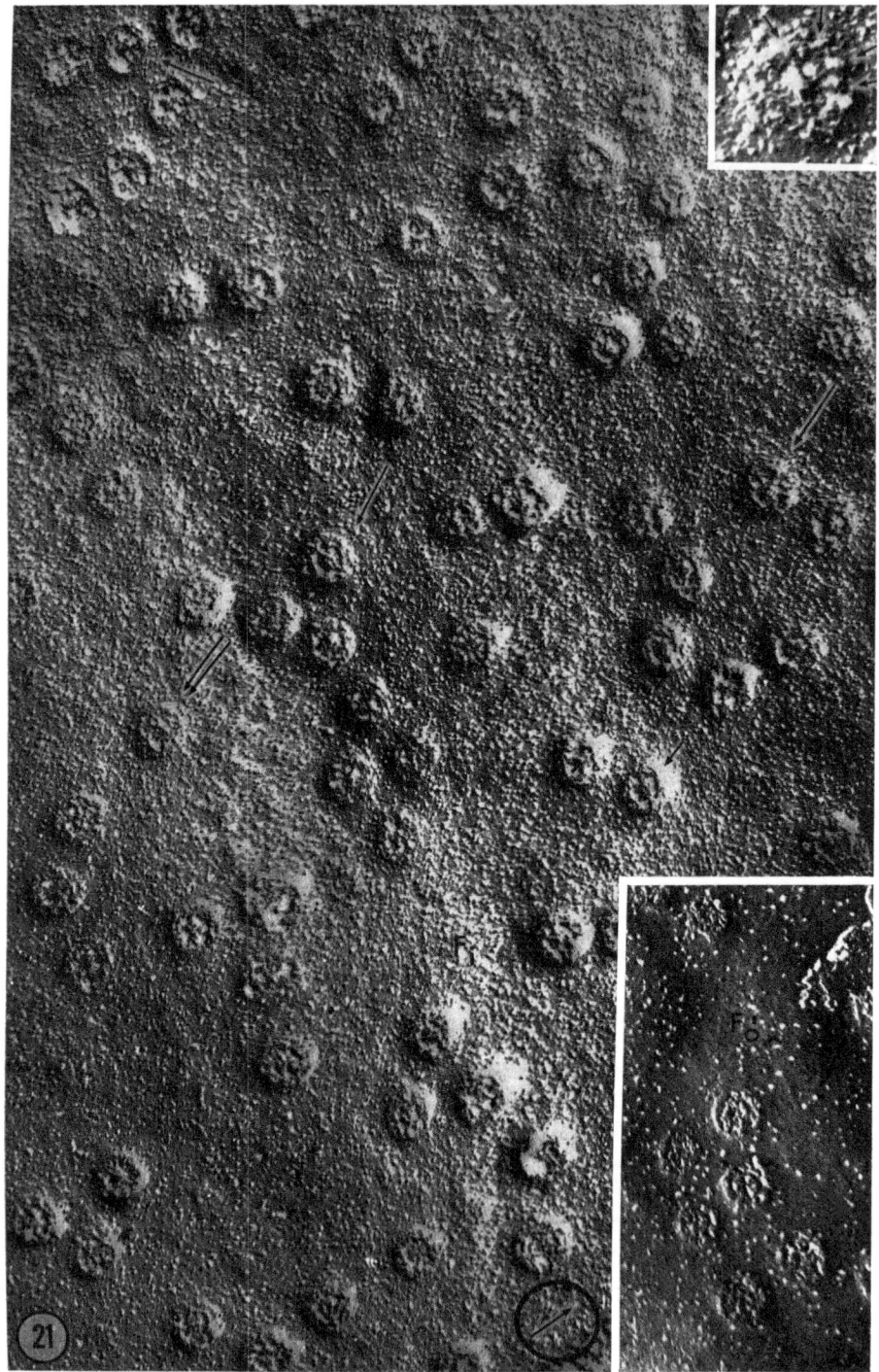

Fig. 21

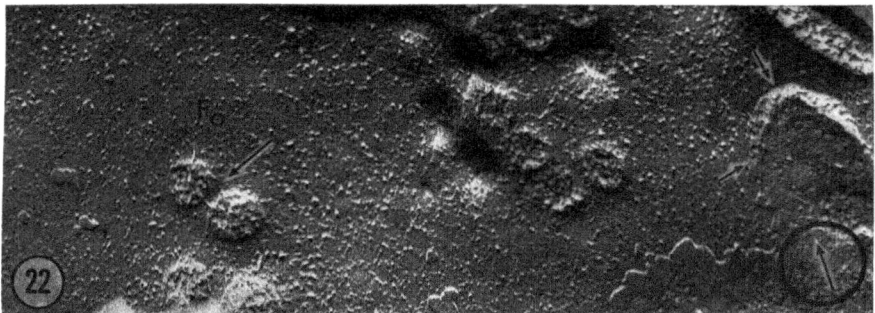

Fig. 22. Concave fracture of a *Pleurochrysis* nuclear envelope. At the transition from the F'_i plane to F_0 an intermediate rim is suggested (arrows in the right) which should correspond to the E_{oc} surface. Note the fibrillar material seemingly connecting adjacent pores. Small islets of the smoother "prime"-fracture plane are visible. Magnification, 61 000:1

might be very poor. Moreover, we have the impression that the type of distribution of these particles is not very meaningful. In course of the present study there were sometimes areas found in the same fracture plane showing a grouping-together of such particles, occasionally with a certain regular arrangement, whereas other areas showed fewer particles. This diversity of particle distribution within one and the same fractured membrane might be another argument against the general use of such freeze-etch particles as spezific morphological membrane markers (compare, e.g., the divergent literature: Remsen *et al.*, 1967; Staehelin, 1968b; Matile and Moor, 1968; Meyer and Winkelmann, 1969; Fill and Branton, 1969; Holt and Stern, 1970; Tillack *et al.*, 1970a and b; Davy and Branton, 1970; Daemer *et al.*, 1970; Fineran, 1970a).

3. Substructural Details of the Pore Complexes

From the afore described observation, that either nuclear membrane tends to be split by the freeze-cleaving process and thus exhibits aspects of the membrane interior, it is easy to understand that in the vast majority of cases the annular subunits (for nomenclature see Franke, 1970; Franke and Scheer, 1970) are splintered away together with the outermost membrane leaflet and thus do not

Fig. 21. Same material as with Fig. 5; a convex fracture of the nuclear envelope. Nuclear pores can be visualized in all fracture faces. For example, the survey shows them in a "non-prime" face of the inner membrane, whereas the insert presents the "prime" face of the outer membrane. The F_i plane is abundant in "particles". Some pore complexes appear as elevated stumps (e.g. the three arrows in the right) according to the fracture scheme of Fig. 26c), whereas others show different aspects including such corresponding to the fracture profile of Fig. 26e (e.g. at the double arrow). Pores suggesting a fracture as sketched under 26b are seen in the upper left (e.g. at the uppermost arrow). Frequently, substructures of the pore interior are resolved, such as the central granule (e.g. at the short arrow in the right) and the radiating fibrils (the uppermost arrow and the upper insert). A structure resembling the inner ring is also sometimes recognized. Magnification, 66000:1; lower insert, 63000:1; upper insert, 135000:1

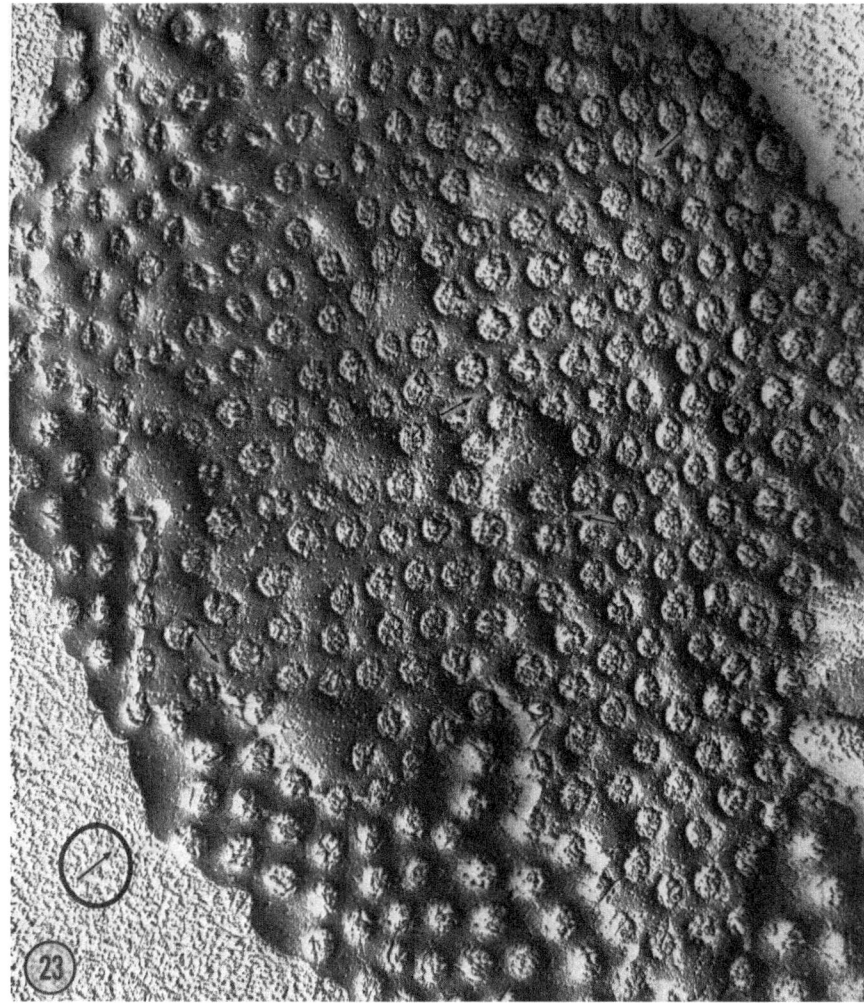

Fig. 23. Fractured nuclear envelope of an intact *Xenopus laevis* lampbrush oocyte. The two fracture faces can be distinguished: a "smooth" one (in the lower part and in the left) interpreted as a "prime" face, and the "non-prime" face which is studded with the particles. Note the high pore frequency. Arrows denote fibrils which seem to "connect" adjacent pore complexes. Magnification, 50000:1

appear in the replica. This was first noted by Franke (1966) and then confirmed by other authors (e.g., Stevens and Andre, 1969; Speth and Wunderlich, 1970; compare, e.g., also Roberts and Northcote, 1970). In a few lucky situations, however, it can apparently happen that the fracture line leaves the membrane interior and jumps over the whole or at least a considerable part of the pore complex proper (e.g. Fig. 26 g–h).[4] In such infrequent situations the

---

[4] For the somewhat similar problems with the freeze-etch appearance of the membrane-attached polysomes the reader is referred to the recent article of Wartiovaara and Branton (1970).

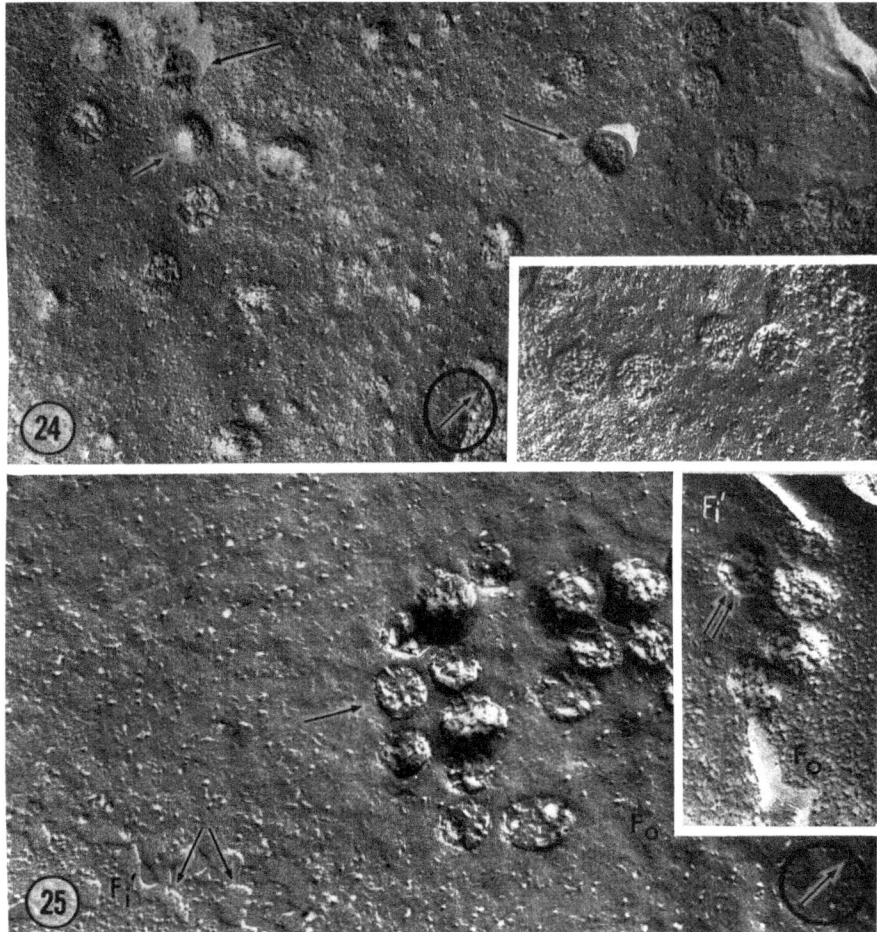

Fig. 24. Frozen-fractured nuclear envelope of the marine alga *Pleurochrysis scherffelii* showing a "non-prime" fracture face. Some pore complexes stand up as prominent cylinders (e.g. at the arrows) whereas others appear as indentations (e.g. at the small arrow in the left). Another category of pores does not show marked relief structures and appears to be filled with a homogeneous "ground-substance" (insert of Fig. 24). Magnification, 34000:1; insert, 59000:1

Fig. 25. Concave nuclear envelope fracture of the same material as presented in the previous figure. In some areas of the nuclear envelope the pores appear clustered together whereas other areas are totally devoid of pores. Islets of a "prime" fracture face (F'_i) stand upon the "non-prime" face of the other nuclear membrane. Within the nuclear pores structural details such as projecting tips (upper arrow) and "inner ring" fibrils (arrows in the insert) are recognized. Magnification, 66000:1; insert, 70000:1

annulus material appears to be sculptured on the pore margin, presumably favored by a relatively deep etching (e.g. Figs. 27 and 30). This is consistent with the recent observation of Roberts and Northcote (1970) of the occurrence of so-called "capped pores" in frozen-etched plant nuclei. Such granular components of the annulus can also be detected in Hess' (1968) micrographs of the

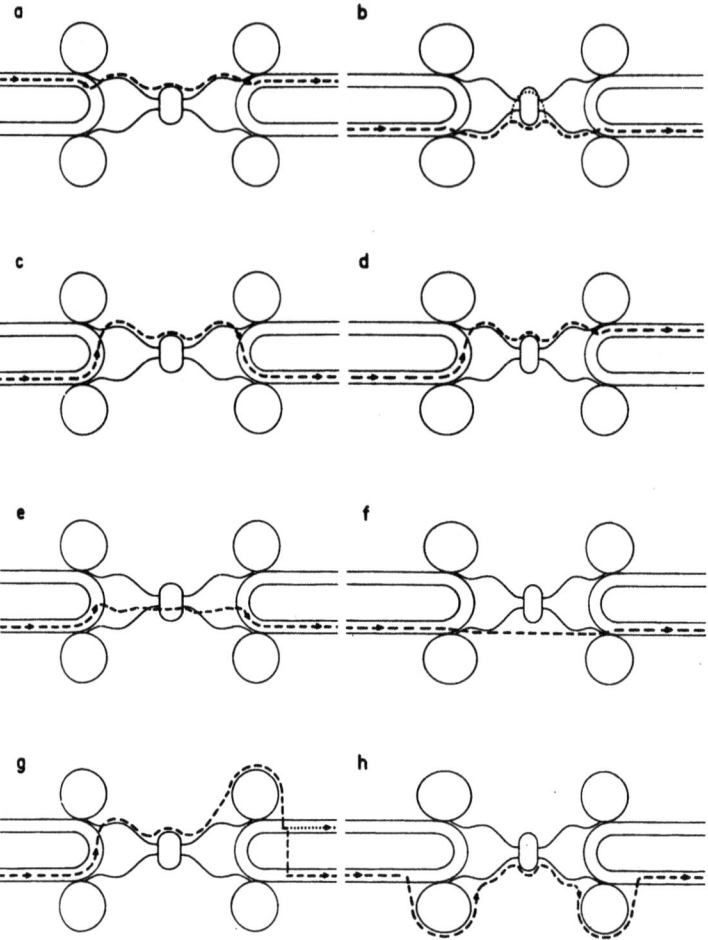

Fig. 26 a–h. Schematic interpretation of some different aspects of the nuclear pore complex as can be revealed after the fracturing (cleaving) process. The fracture line can leave the membrane when a certain angle of inclination with the anticlinal pore walls is attained (f), thus giving a rise to the appearence of holes with a diameter more or less larger than the true inner pore diameter[5] and re-enter either the same side or the other side of the nuclear membrane. It may also follow the curvature of the pore wall for a certain distance, then leave the membrane and re-enter the same-sided membrane at the other side of the pore, thereby jumping over the dense components of the pore interior such as the projecting tips, the inner pore fibrils and the central granule: the different types of relief which can be produced by such fracturing are shown in Fig. a–c. A variant of this type is the straight fracturing through the pore complex material (e). On the other hand, it can happen that the fracture line does not continue in the same side of the nuclear membrane but changes over to the other side of the membrane as indicated in Fig. d. Fracture lines which leave the membrane relatively early and jump over the non-membraneous pore complex material including the annulus (Fig. h) are relatively seldom (compare the "capped pores" of Roberts and Northcote, 1970) whereas fracture lines which round and sculpture only parts of an annulus (g) are more frequently observed.

---

[5] i.e. the luminal width in the equatorial plane of the pore.

frozen-etched fungus Pyrenochaeta terrestris. Both conceivable types of annular subunits appearance, i.e. either as elevations corresponding to the case depicted in Fig. 26g or as indentations as sketched in Fig. 26 h could be found, and both showed the typical eightfold radial symmetry of distribution demonstrated earlier from negatively stained isolated envelope fragments (Franke, 1966, 1967; Gall, 1967; Franke and Kartenbeck, 1969; Comes and Franke, 1970; Franke and Scheer, 1970a) as well as from thin sections (Fisher and Cooper, 1967; Bajer and Molé-Bajer, 1969; Daniels et al., 1969; de Zoeten and Gaard, 1969; Franke, 1970). This eightfold radial symmetry is, for example, documented in Fig. 33 by Markham's rotation technique of a Pleurochrysis scherffelii pore complex in which the annular subunits appear as indentations. This aspect can also be found in a great many micrographs of the literature. So, e.g., some of the pores shown in the micrograph figure F-2 (onion root tip cells; Branton and Moor, 1964) presented in Frey-Wyssling and Mühlethaler's book (1965) exhibit a precise eight-point radial symmetry when examined with the technique of Markham et al. (1963).

Today's literature on frozen-etched biomembranes does not show many examples of situations related to the demonstration of the membrane-associated annulus material. One is the afore-cited investigation of Wartiovaara and Branton (1970) on the appearance of membrane-attached ribosomes. Another example appears to be the work of Bracker and Grove (1970). These authors showed regularly spaced, distinct $50-80 \times 120-180$ Å knobs as being apposed to the outer mitochondrial membrane of the oomycetous fungus Pythium ultimum with both thin sectioning and freeze-etch technique: This presentation thus at least makes clear that membrane-associated particles, presumably of a proteinaceous nature, can in some manner be sculptured on frozen-cleaved membrane faces.

Combining all aspects obtained in the present study the appearance of frozen etched nuclear pores can be the result of one of the fracture possibilities sketched in Fig. 26. For example, a fracture line within either of the nuclear membranes can follow the curvature at the pore rim for a certain distance, then, where approaching the pore-equator, it leaves the membrane and runs either straight through the inner pore material (Fig. 26e) or follows the profile of the inner pore constituents such as the projecting tip material and the centrale granule. Subsequently, it can continue within the nuclear membrane of the same side (Fig. 26a–c) or may change over to the other (Fig. 26d). Replicas of such fractures through pore complexes usually reveal the pore margin as a more or less sharply outlined demarcation circumscribing the projecting tips, which can be attached to the pore wall as described from other techniques (see Franke, 1970), and the central granule[6]. These latter two compact structures, consequently, can be recognized in some of the preparations as elevated particles or as indentations in the pore complex "ground-substance" (e.g., Figs. 25, 27, 29, 31, 32, 34). On the other hand, in the cases where the fracture runs straight through the pore interior and/or where the etching was non-sufficient the pores seem to be filled by more or less coarsely textured "ground-substance" alone (Moor and Mühle-

---

[6] The central granule can be readily recognized in most studies of frozen-etched nuclei (e.g., Frey-Wyssling and Mühlethaler, 1965; Hess, 1968; Northcote and Lewis, 1968; Speth and Wunderlich, 1970).

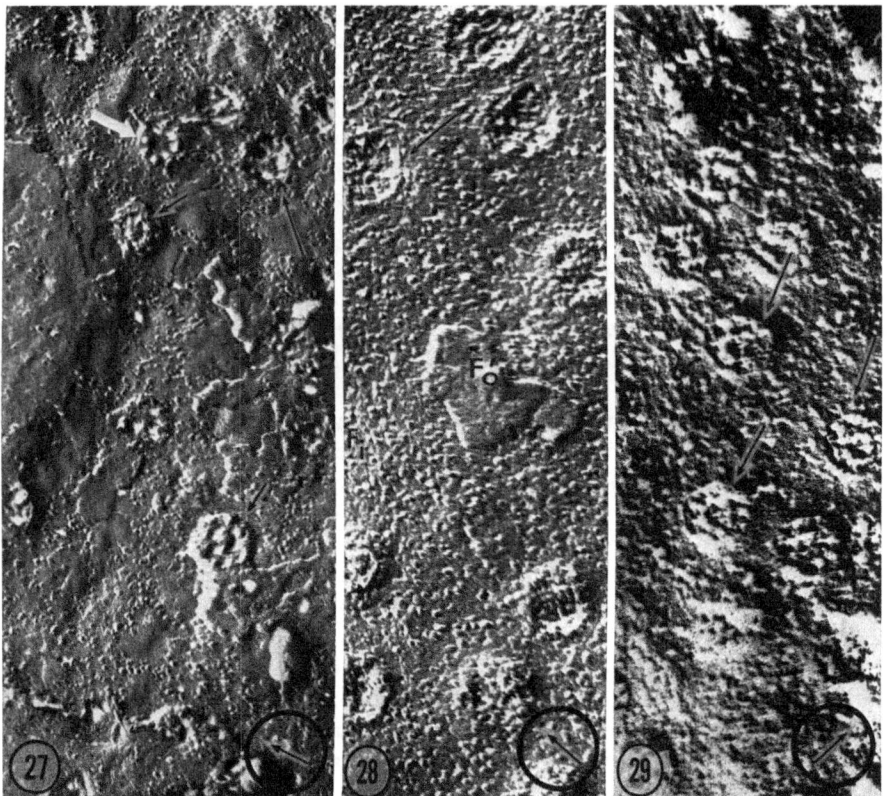

Figs. 27–29. Same material as with Fig. 5. Details of freeze-etch aspects of fractured nuclear pore complexes. The diversity of the fracturing of the pore complex can be seen from Fig. 27. The short arrows denote a situation in which the annulus material appears to be preserved and which resembles the fracture described under Fig. 26g. The long arrows in the right points to a pore complex which seemingly has been fractured as sketched in Fig. 26b. The white arrow indicates a pore complex fracture with the "projecting tips" at the inner pore wall as elevated structures, according to the interpretation of Fig. 26c. A situation interpreted as representing the case shown in Fig. 26f is recognized with the majority of the pores of Fig. 28 (e.g. at the arrow). The "non-prime" envelope fracture plane of Fig. 29 shows a conspicuous predominance of the case of Fig. 26a with prominent projecting tips in the pore interior.
Fig. 27, 72000:1; Figs. 28 and 29, 90000:1

thaler, 1963; see e.g., Figs. 21–24, 28). Frequently, the typical "inner fibrils" of the pore complex could be visualized in the frozen-etched pores as being either radially oriented, sometimes raying out from the central granule, or as arranged in the form of the "inner ring" (e.g., Figs. 21 and 25). Occasionally, similar filaments were seen to connect two adjacent pore complexes (e.g., Fig. 22): these latter, however, should then represent filamentous material within the membrane rather than lying on the membrane. Such pore-complex associated fibrils have also been reported by Maul (1970).

An especially interesting system with respect to the nuclear pore complex subarchitecture is the bird erythrocyte. With this cell type, thin sections as well

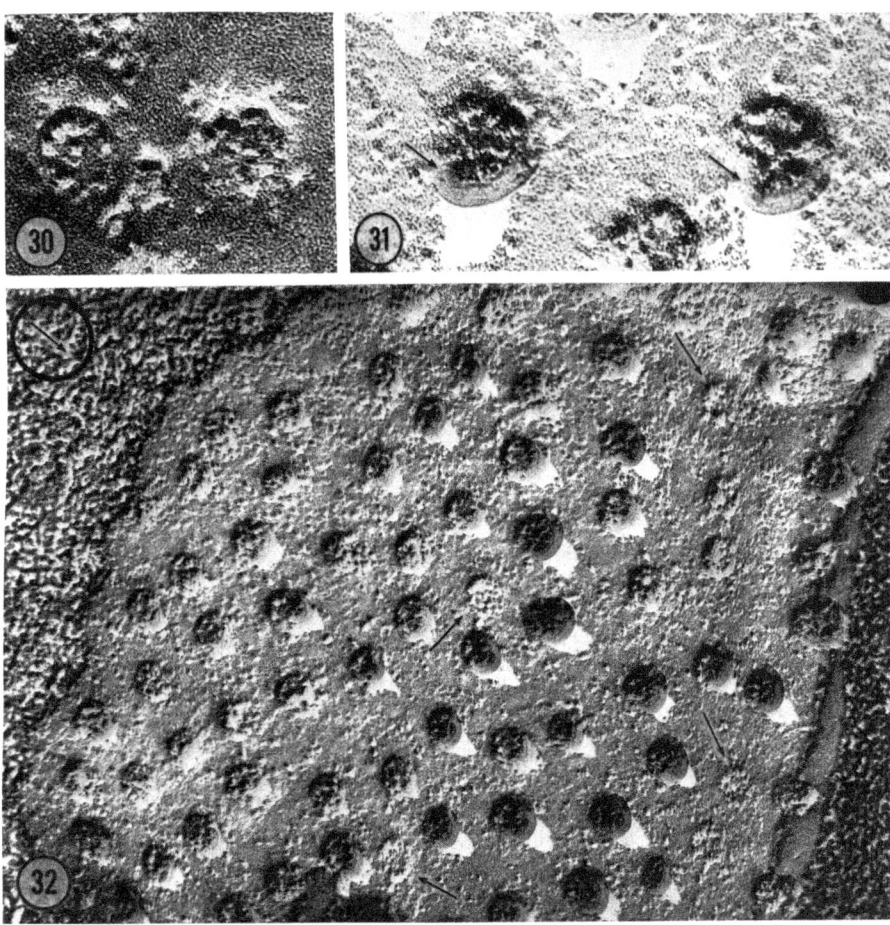

Figs. 30 and 31. Appearance of pore complexes of the *Triturus* oocytes in detail. Fig. 31 represents a fracture corresponding to Fig. 26g: the pore circumference (arrows) is partly covered by the annular granules. The pores shown in Fig. 41 are interpreted as representing the case of Fig. 26a: the projecting tips protrude from the pore wall into the lumen. A central granule is clearly seen. Both figures, 160000:1

Fig. 32. Nucleus isolated from a mature Alpine newt oocyte, previously fixed with 2% glutaraldehyde, incubated in glycerol and frozen-etched. Many of the pore complexes stand upon the particle set "non-prime" fracture face as compact cylinders as indicated by their long shadows. It can not be excluded, though, that remnants of biological material, for which has not been washed off with the chromic acid, contribute to these stumps. In the contrary, other adjacent pores are hardly identified (arrows). This might be a consequence of a fracture according to the case sketched in Fig. 26e. Note the "prime face" at the left margin. Magnification, 64000:1

as negatively stained preparations did not show either the presence of annulus material nor fibrils within the pore; the only substructures seen in thin sections is a dense "diaphragm-like" matter in the very pore equator. With freeze-etching these nuclei also did not reveal such pore substructures. They usually appeared

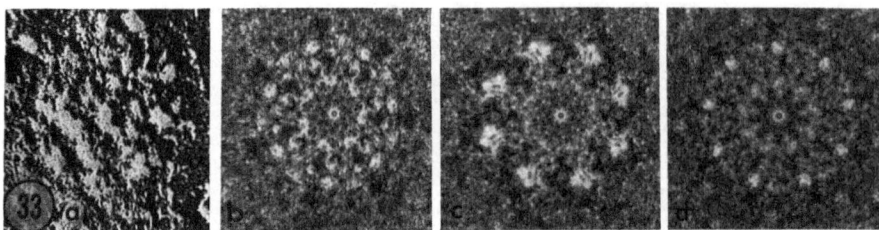

Fig. 33a–d. Markham Analysis of a *Pleurochrysis* nuclear pore complex cross fractured in a mode related to that indicated in Fig. 26h. The pattern of annular granules, which here appear as indentations, is reinforced at $n=8$ (c) and not at $n=7$ (b) and $n=9$ (d). Magnification, 160000:1

to be filled with the amorphous ground substance (e.g., Fig. 2), the only detail suggested in a few cases being a compact ring at the inner pore wall (Fig. 39).

Cross-fractures of the anticlinal pore walls (Fig. 35) sometimes can be resolved to demonstrate a "dark-light-dark" appearance (distance 50 Å) which, according to the fracture schemes of Fig. 26a–e, should correspond to approximately half a unit membrane. The width of this triple-structure is significantly below that of the total membrane, a finding which is in accordance with our interpretation of the fracturing (see Fig. 35). In agreement with the study of Roberts and Northcote (1970) we emphasize our earlier view that the normal outline of the pores proper is circular, as this is especially conspicuous with Pleurochrysis (e.g., Fig. 35), in which stabilizing or ice crystal preventing treatment was not necessary. Deviations from circularity might have been artificially caused (for more detailed discussions see also Franke, 1967; Northcote and Lewis, 1968; Franke, 1970; Franke and Scheer, 1970; Maul, 1970).

Another also less frequently observed fracture line concluded from our micrographs is depicted in Fig. 26 g: Probably as a consequence of the high physical density of the inner pore material (about 1.35–1.55 in comparison with the 1.16–1.21 of the nuclear membrane itself, e.g., Kashnig and Kasper, 1969; Zbarsky et al., 1969; Franke et al., 1970; Zentgraf et al., 1971) the fracture leaves the membrane, sculptures the inner pore material, jumps around part of the annulus and finally enters the membrane again. This fracturing behaviour suggests a high stability and rigidity of the non-membranous pore complex material as indicated from the fragmentation behaviour (e.g., Fig. 40; see also Monroe et al., 1967; Yoo and Bayley, 1967; Franke and Kartenbeck, 1969; Scheer and Franke, 1969; Scheer, 1970). The characteristic picture of the pore complex thus fractured is a short column-like stump with a more or less irregular height (e.g., Figs. 24, 28, 32). The maximal height of this stump is necessarily in the order of the width of the perinuclear cisterna. Very frequently this specific aspect of pore complex fracturing varied from pore to pore even though the underlying membrane fracture face appeared basically to be continuous; this is especially demonstrated, e.g., in Figs. 21, 23, 24, 32 and 34.

It should perhaps be stressed that all the basic pore complex constituents described from other techniques are not only seen in frozen-etched material after

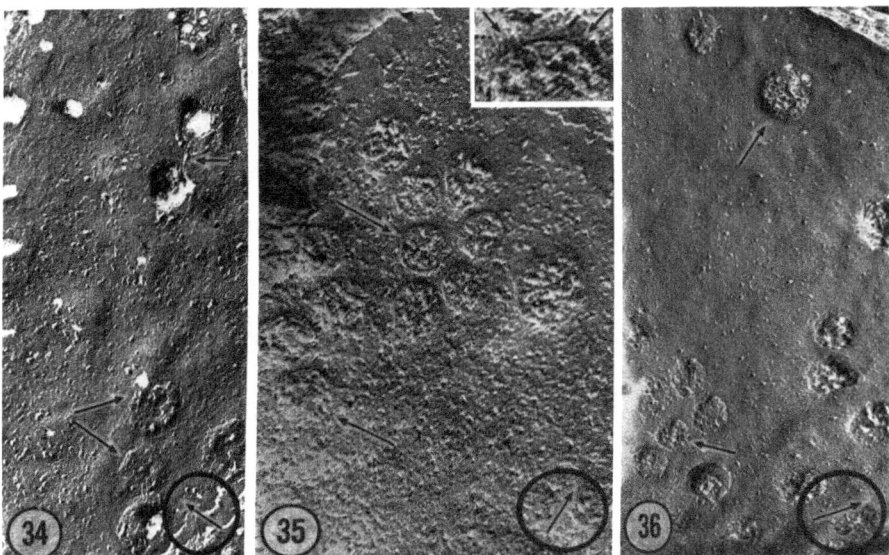

Figs. 34–36. Details of frozen-fractured nuclear pore complexes of *Pleurochrysis*. The "non-prime" faces sometimes show prominent ring-like structures (Fig. 34) which suggest pores but can not clearly identified (lower arrows). A fibril extending between adjecent "pore-holes" is denoted by the upper small arrow. The pore diameter is best recognized in cross-fractured pore complexes (Fig. 35). Occasionally, cross fractured pore walls can be resolved in a 50–60 Å broad dark-light-dark triple-layer pattern which then should correspond to approximately half-a-membrane according to the fracture scheme of Fig. 26e. The size of the holes in the fractured nuclear envelope vary widely (Fig. 36, arrows). Probably the larger holes reflect situations caused by a fracturing indicated in the scheme Fig. f. Fig. 34, 68000:1; Fig. 35, 66000:1; inset of Fig. 35, 130000:1; Fig. 36, 50000:1

prestabilization and incubation in anti-crystallization agents, but also in the example of Pleurochrysis in which no fixation and glycerol treatment is needed.

It is also conceivable that the fracture does not leave the nuclear membrane at the very sites of the pore circumference, but leaves the membrane more or less before that as this is sketched in Fig. 3f. This is particularly likely with those nuclear envelopes in which the two nuclear membranes have an especially high tendency to converge upon the pore equator under a relatively low angle. Such a rupture line would then reveal a "hole" within the membrane face which corresponds to the existence of a pore in this area, but is not an image of the pore structure itself. Such "pore corresponding rupture holes" would simulate "true nuclear pores" since they appear filled with a homogeneous ground-substance that actually, however, is either cyto- or nucleoplasm[7]. A rupture line of this kind would also provide a straightforward explanation of the observation of "pores" with exceedingly large diameters, as have been consistently observed throughout the present study, in particular with the hen erythro-

_____

[7] That such a pore-filling ground-substance is not a special freeze-etch aspect of a cellular component might best be seen from its appearance within the endothelial fenestrae (Wisse, 1970).

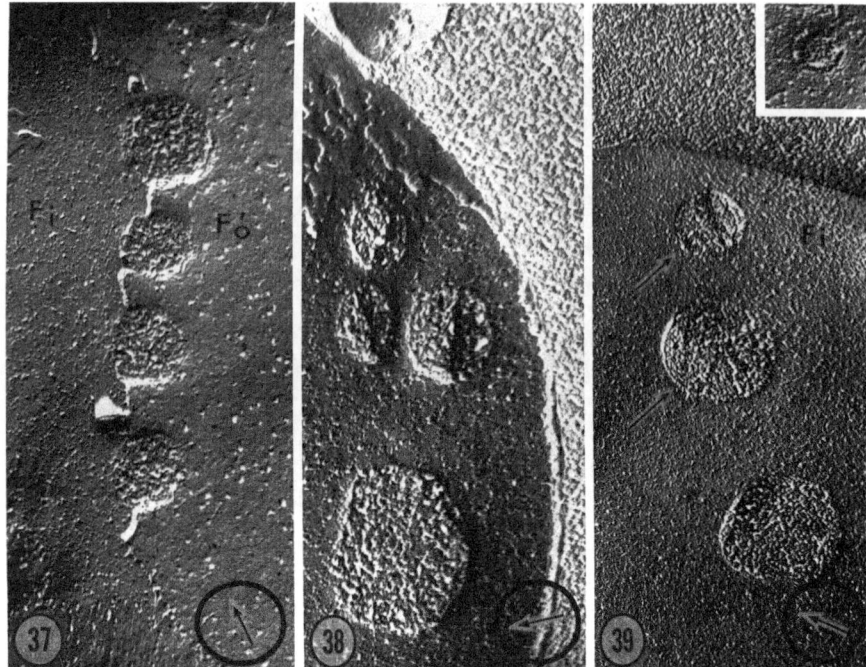

Figs. 37–39. Details of frozen-etched pore complexes of hen erythrocyte nuclei. At the nuclear pores the fracture shows a particularly high tendency to change from the fracture face of one nuclear membrane to that of the other (Fig. 37). The wide range of the diameters of fracture holes in the nuclear envelope, be they pores or not, is demonstrated in the other two micrographs and is especially clear from comparing the adjacent pores marked by the arrows in Fig. 39. The only structural detail ever observed in the interior of the frozen-etched nuclear pores in this cell is a ring of material protruding from the pore circumference into the pore lumen (insert of Fig. 39). Fig. 37, 55000:1; Fig. 38, 68000:1; Fig. 39, 42000:1

cytes and Pleurochrysis scherffelii. Extremely large "pores" have also been reported from freeze-etch studies with various other systems (e.g., Branton and Moor, 1964). It is contradictory to the results obtained from thin section electron microscopy and generally hard to imagine that adjacent pores can vary in diameter from, e.g., 1300 to 3500 Å as presented in Figs. 38 and 39. A similar case is documented for Pleurochrysis in Fig. 36. The somewhat bimodal distribution of the "apparent pore sizes" found with the hen erythrocytes would at least be easily explained by such a mixed population of true pores and artificial "pore corresponding holes". In addition to the occurrence of the artificial holes produced by the rupturing indicated in Fig. 26f the general possibility cannot be excluded that holes may be produced in areas where a nuclear pore does not exist in that a fracture cuts off localized blebs and other sorts of natural or artificial evaginations or cuts through the cisternal connections with the endoplasmic reticulum (ER). Blebbing of vesicles from, e.g., the outer nuclear envelope is documented for many cell systems as well as is the ER-continuity. On the other hand, we would like to attach particular importance to the general observation that clearly recognizable pores could be seen in a given nuclear envelope area just beside others, which were hardly recognizable. Moreover certain structures could be seen in a nuclear envelope in which we could not tell whether this is a pore or not (e.g. Figs. 32 and 34). Such findings strongly suggest that nuclear pores may not be a priori identifiable in a frozen-etched nuclear envelope.

4. Arrangement of Pores

Nuclear pores are relatively equally distributed on the nuclear surfaces of the rat hepatocytes and hen erythrocytes, and basically also with the amphibian oocytes, whereas Pleurochrysis is somewhat different. Here a pronounced tendency of clusters of pores grouped together was found (e.g. Fig. 25). Such a grouping of nuclear pores has been mentioned earlier from diverse cell systems (e.g., Northcote and Lewis, 1968), especially from some Dinoflagellates (Wecke and Giesbrecht, 1970). With all the objects of this study nuclear envelope areas could be seen without pores, besides others which where abundant in pores, but this nevertheless could still represent a random distribution. It is especially worth emphasizing that with the amphibian oocytes the ordered densely packed pore arrangements known from other techniques were observed also in the freeze-etching (Fig. 23). In addition, however, occasionally nuclear envelope areas almost devoid of pores were also met (e.g. Fig. 41). There is no obvious explanation for the above mentioned clustering existing in the envelopes of some cell types (compare e.g. the discussion on the "closed", "open" and "forming" pores in Frey-Wyssling and Mühlethaler, 1965; Maul, 1970).

5. Quantitative Structural Data: A Methodical Comparison

Structural data of the nuclear envelope, such as the pore diameter and the pore frequency (pores per square micron), can differ in the same material according to the specific electron microscopic methods used (thin sectioning, negative staining of isolated nuclear envelope fragments, freeze-etching) as has been noted as early as 1966 (Franke, 1966; see also Franke, 1970). The average pore diameter appears significantly larger with the freeze-etch process and the pore frequency is usually much lower. In our laboratory a methodical comparison was attempted in order to elucidate these perplexing observations. The increase of the pore frequency in the sequence: freeze-etching of whole cells → thin section preparations of whole cells → negative staining of the isolated nuclear envelope fragments as well as a corresponding decrease in pore diameter values has been recently confirmed by Speth and Wunderlich (1970) with the ciliate Tetrahymena pyriformis GL macronucleus.

When one quantitatively evaluates the dimensions of the nuclear envelope one has always to keep in mind the possible sources of error as are indicated from the previous chapter. So, for instance, fractures through pore complexes do not necessarily demonstrate the true pore diameter but rather tend to produce the "pore corresponding holes" according to the fracturing shown in Fig. 26f. Consequently, in the present authors' opinion, a good deal of measurements of pore diameters in freeze-etch micrographs as given in the literature are likely to refer to a mixed population consisting of images of pores and of such "pore corresponding holes". In addition to that, it is a consequence of the low resolution obtained with the present days' shadowing procedure (for future aspects see Bachmann et al., 1969) that the precision of measuring a pore diameter cannot be better than ± 50 Å, i.e. about 7% of the pore size (see however, also Easterbrook and Rozee, 1971).

Moreover, with respect to pore frequencies one has to be aware of the above indicated possibilities that a certain number of pores are not revealed by the freeze-etch technique: a pore counting in areas like, e.g., that shown in Fig. 23 thus might result in pore frequency values which are too low.

(a) Pleurochrysis scherffelii. The mean pore diameter after freeze-etching was 116 ± 7 nm. This value is about 35% higher than the average value obtained from thin sections through cells fixed with glutaraldehyde in situ (Brown and Franke, unpublished).

(b) Hen erythrocytes. The diameter of all "holes which suggest a correspondence to nuclear pores" was at an average of 167 nm. This is in strong contrast to the diameters measured from thin section electron micrographs (mean value: 70 nm) and from negatively stained isolated envelope fragments (61 nm). This difference seems to be caused, at least partially, by the hole producing fracture lines around the pore mentioned above (Fig. 26f). The pore frequency determinations revealed values fairly agreeing, namely 3 ± 1 pores/μ^2 (freeze-etching) and 4 ± 1 pores/μ^2 (thin sections). A determination of the pore frequencies from the isolated envelope fragements did not make sense since these fragments were too small and seldom contained more than 1 to 3 pores (compare Zentgraf et al., 1971).

(c) Rat liver cells. The quantitative evaluation of the nuclear envelope of the rat liver parenchymal cells is presented in table I. Here again the pore diameter appears to be larger with the freeze-etching preparation of the tissue (prestabilized with glutaraldehyde) than with the tissue processed for thin section electron microscopy and, even more, with the isolated nuclear envelope fragments. In order to find out during which preparation step such changes in pore diameter could have taken place three other preparations were evaluated. Franke (1970) has conjectured that the changes in nuclear envelope structure observed with the isolated nuclear envelope pieces could be the result of the fragmentation process as such: reduction of nuclear, and possibly also intracisternal, turgor leads to a cisternal shrinkage (compare also Speth and Wunderlich, 1970).

It has been known for a long time that nuclei of diverse plant and animal cell types tend to undergo a dramatic shrinkage when isolation procedures using hypertonic sucrose are applied, especially in the presence of bivalent cations (e.g. Anderson and Wilbur, 1952; Accola, 1960). So Accola (1960) has reported the diameter of onion root tip nuclei isolated in ca. 2,3 M sucrose to shrink by 30% or even more. Since the envelopes of such isolated nuclei usually exhibit frequent sites of interruption it is not yet clear whether shrinkage of nuclear diameter necessarily must be correlated with shrinkage of the nuclear envelope area (for some experimental results relevant to this problem see also the subsequent chapter on the amphibian oocytes). Furthermore, with respect to the mechanisms of such alterations in nuclear morphology, it has to be kept

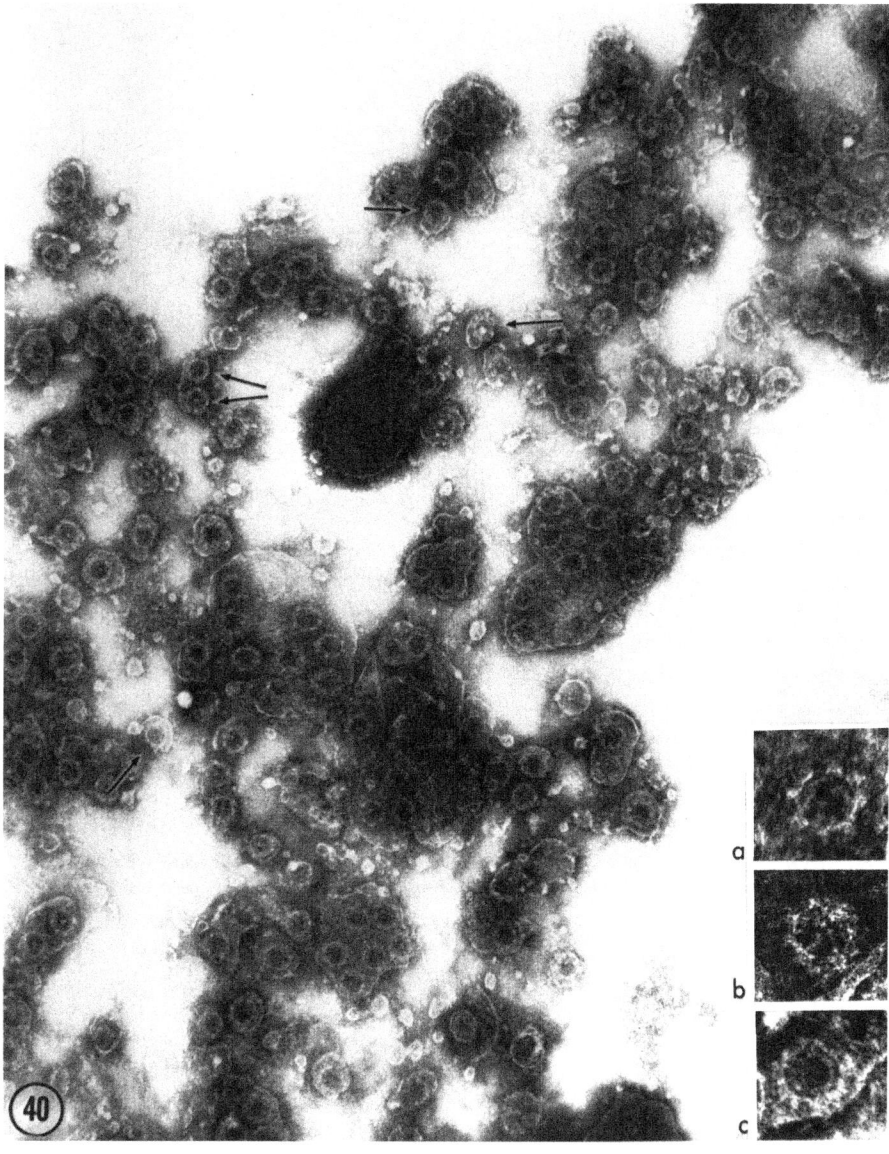

Fig. 40a–c. Negatively stained (PTA) fraction of purified nuclear envelope fragments isolated from rat liver. Note the variation in fragmental sizes. The fragmentation lines tend to run around the pore complexes (arrows), thus indicating the mechanical stability of the pore complexes. Pore complex substructures such as central granules with varying diameters (e.g. at the arrows), annular particles (e.g. insert a), radiating filaments (insert b), and the "inner ring" (insert c) can frequently be recognized. Magnification, 39000:1; insert a–c, 100000:1

in mind that such shrinkage primarily reflects the condensation of the chromatinous mass, and that thus it is the "precipitated" state of the chromatin which maintains the specific nuclear morphology (for the particular clear

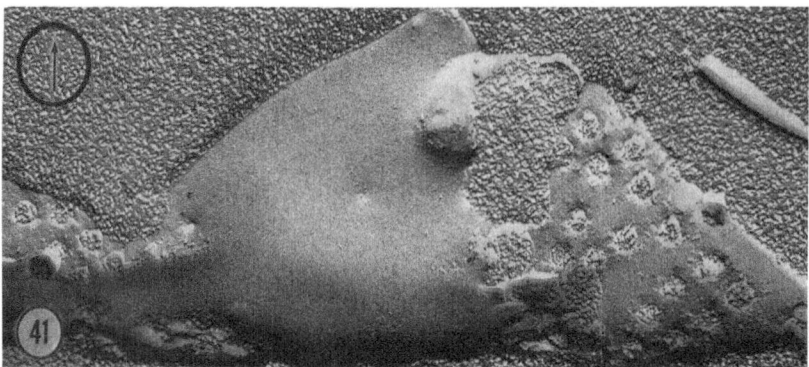

Fig. 41. Part of a nuclear envelope of an isolated, aldehyde and glycerol treated freeze-etched nucleus of a *Triturus alpestris* oocyte. Areas with pores can be seen beside relatively large regions which do not bear pores. Magnification, 43000:1

example of the muscle nucleus see, e.g., Franke and Schinko, 1969; Schinko, 1970). It is altogether conceivable that the interphase nuclear envelope which is tightly linked to the chromatin by the anchoring pieces of the nuclear DNA in its interporous areas (for references see "Introduction"), just passively follows the chromatin shrinkage by either reducing its own surface area or by rupturing.

This view of nuclear surface shrinkage is not supported by measurements of pore diameters among the envelope pieces of widely varying fragment sizes (e.g. Fig. 40): the pore diameter does not change proportionally to the fragment size. Neither does the "nuclear envelope shrinkage hypothesis" hold for explaining the reduction in pore diameter as taking place in the course of isolation and fragmentation of the nucleus. There is also no support for this view from the measurements of the pore diameter of the isolated nuclei with the other preparation methods, i.e. thin section and freeze-etching techniques (e.g. Figs. 42 and 43). On the other hand, a comparison of the pore diameter values as according to the different procedures strongly suggests that the appearance of larger pore diameters is due to the freeze-etching technique as such and probably reflects the diverse fissures around the pores already mentioned (compare Fig. 26) which give rise to "pseudo-pore-diameters" and which are necessarily larger than the true pore diameters. The "balloon hypothesis" (Franke, 1970) has also been discussed to provide an explanation for the increase of pores per surface unit, which is observed in the methods employed as quoted above. This concept was somewhat supported by the remark of Bajer and Mole-Bajer (1969) that during the break-down of the nuclear envelope in the prometaphase of mitosis in the blood lily endosperm, the number of pores per square micron increases from 20–25 to 38–42, which effect these authors also described to a contraction of the perinuclear cisternal fragment. The pore frequency measurements listed in table I clearly demonstrate that, in fact, the number of pores per square micron increases when the nucleus is isolated. This would be fairly in line with a nuclear envelope shrinkage explanation during the homogenization and isolation steps.

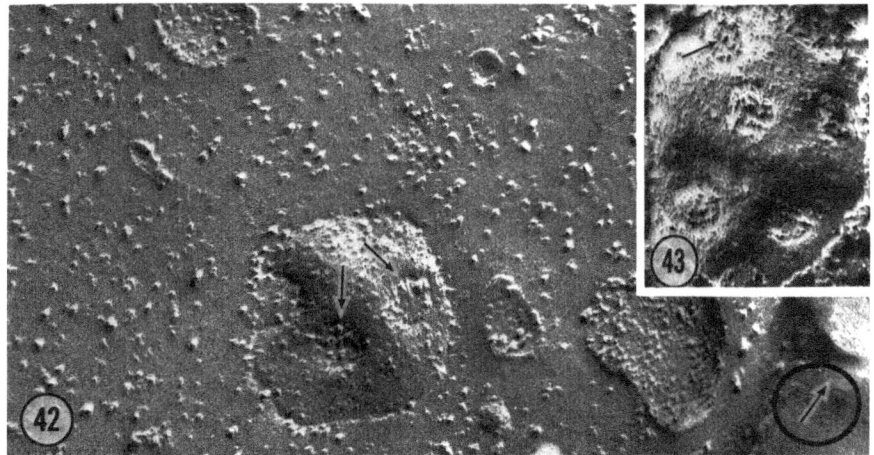

Figs. 42 and 43. Freeze-etching preparation of nuclear envelope fragments isolated from rat liver. Nuclear pores can be identified but show somewhat varying aspects (compare Fig. 42 and 43). Note that many "freeze-etch particles" can be seen which are definitely not associated with membranes but appear "free" on the frozen medium. Fig. 42: arrows indicate nuclear pores; Fig. 43: arrow indicates a central granule. Both figures, 80000:1

Table 1. Structural data of the nuclear envelope of rat liver cells as revealed after the different electron microscopic preparation techniques

Type of preparation	Nuclear pores/μm^2	Pore diameter (nm)
Nuclei in situ, fixed and freeze-etched	14.1 ± 2.3	88 ± 8
Nuclei in situ, fixed, dehydrated, embedded and sectioned	16.3 ± 1.5	68 ± 6
Isolated nuclei, fixed and freeze-etched	24.9 ± 3.0	78 ± 6
Isolated nuclear membranes, fixed and freeze-etched	24.3 ± 7.5	89 ± 7
Isolated nuclear membranes[a] fixed and negatively stained (PTA)	35.8 ± 4.3	67 ± 2

[a] Mean values from fragments larger than 0.3 μm^2.

Further fragmentation might then lead to another increase in pore frequency. Such an increase seems to be especially true in the case of the negative staining preparation (Table 1) and apparently even greater increases occur after high salt extraction treatment (Franke et al., 1970). That the pore frequency is not proportional to the size of the envelope fragments is suggested from the diagram of Fig. 44. Taken together, our measurements lead to the conclusion that the diversity in pore diameter has something to do with the appearance of the nuclear pores in freeze-etch preparations and that the shrinkage processes can cause changes only to a minor degree. On the other hand the pore frequency differences apparently seem to be due to different effects, namely to the nuclear (and nuclear envelope) shrinkage during isolation and fragmentation and possibly also to a specific reaction to the negative staining preparation. These two effects then may

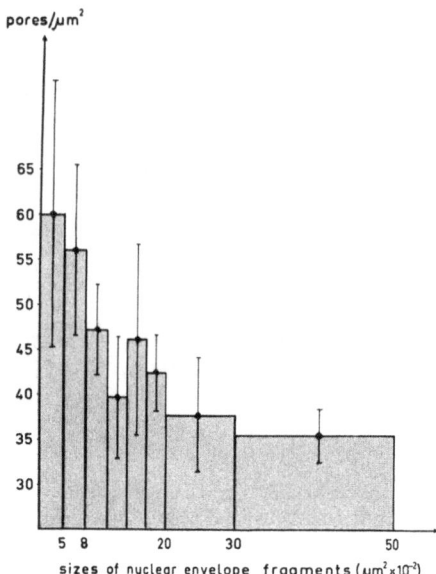

Fig. 44. Correlation between frequency and nuclear envelope fragment size as measured in nuclear membrane fractions isolated from rat liver (compare Fig. 40)

be additive. Furthermore, the measurements indicate that the non pore-bearing perinuclear cisternal area is more labile in terms of shrinking than the pore complex itself. This fits into the view of the pore complex as a structural unit relatively stable against mechanical stress (see Fig. 40 and the previous chapters; compare also Yoo and Bayley, 1967; Monroe et al., 1968; Scheer and Franke, 1969; Franke and Kartenbeck, 1969; Scheer, 1970).

(d) Amphibian oocytes. The nuclear surface of the frozen-etched Xenopus laevis lampbrush oocytes shows the pore complexes in a relatively regular distribution (e.g. Fig. 23). The pore frequency amounted in this stage of oogenesis to 60 ± 4 pores/μ^2. The same value was obtained with and without prefixation of the oocytes with formaldehyde prior to the glycerol incubation (for details see Scheer, 1970). As can be seen from table II, negatively stained isolated nuclear envelopes (Fig. 45), thin sections tangential to nuclei of fixed whole oocytes (e.g. Fig. 46) and to isolated nuclei (e.g. Fig. 47) showed nearly identical pore frequencies with this material. Nuclei isolated from mature Triturus alpestris oocytes revealed almost the same pore frequencies, namely 50 pores per square micron, after freeze-etching technique as well as in negative staining preparations (see also Scheer, 1970).

With respect to pore diameters all the three preparation methods again resulted in nearly identical values (Table 2).

The obvious contrast between the nuclei of the amphibian oocytes and the rat hepatocytes may reflect the specific responses of the nuclear envelopes to the influences during the various electron microscopical preparations. Semi-thin

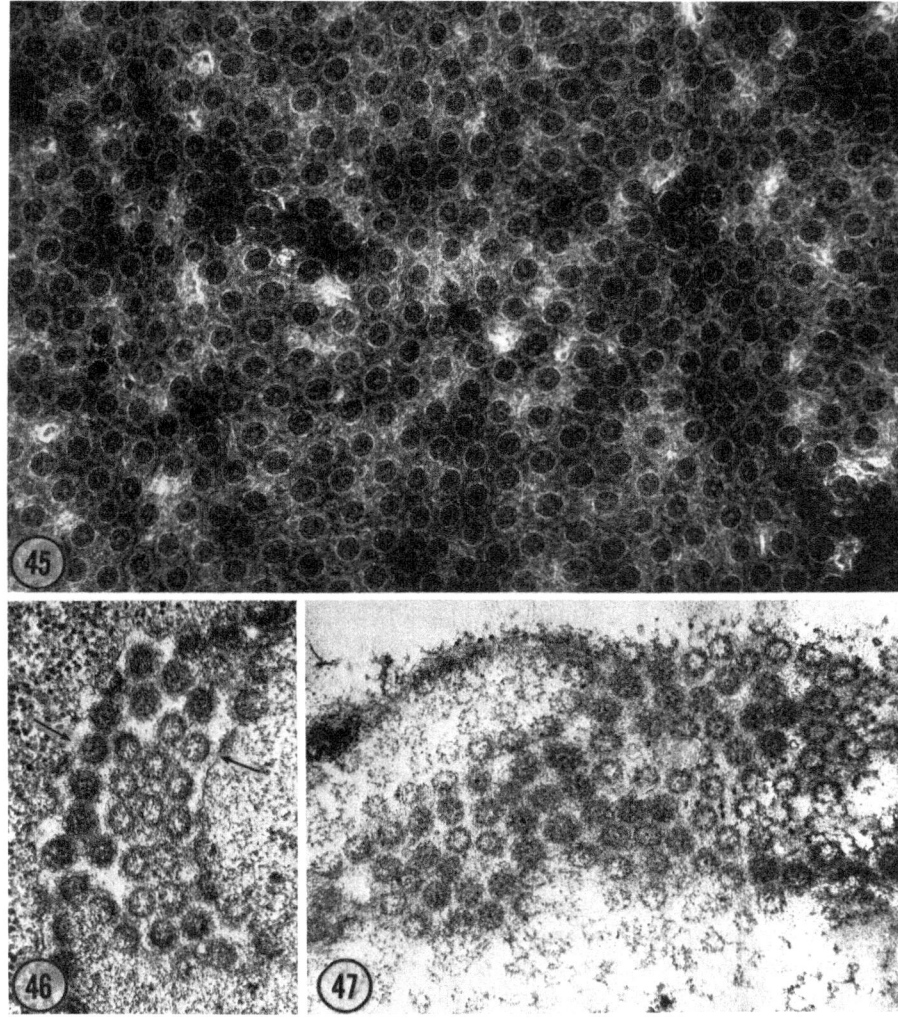

Fig. 45. Negatively stained (2% PTA) nuclear envelope isolated from a lampbrush stage *Xenopus laevis* oocyte. The isolation was carried out in the "5:1-medium" without an addition of stabilizing bivalent cations. In such preparations the pore diameter is clearly visible. Magnification, 40000:1

Fig. 46. Thin section tangential to the nuclear envelope of an intact *Xenopus laevis* lampbrush oocyte. In sections which include the anticlinal pore walls a precise measurement of the pore diameter is possible (arrows). Magnification, 40000:1

Fig. 47. Thin section grazing to a nucleus isolated from a *Xenopus* lampbrush oocyte. Magnification, 40000:1

sections of fixed and Epon-embedded lampbrush oocytes show in the phase contrast microscope a "wrinkling", i.e. an abundance of invaginations and outfoldings of the nuclear envelope, whereas the nuclear border in 10 μ thick

Table 2. *Structural data of the nuclear envelope of lampbrush stage* Xenopus laevis *oocytes (nuclear diameter 520 μm) as revealed after the different electron microscopic preparation techniques*

Type of preparation	Nuclear pores/μm²	Pore diameter (nm)
Nuclei in situ, fixed and freeze-etched	60 ± 4	74.2 ± 3.3
Nuclei in situ, fixed, dehydrated, embedded and sectioned	60 ± 8	71.5 ± 3.1
Isolated nuclei fixed, dehydrated, embedded and sectioned	67 ± 3	73.0 ± 3.1
Isolated nuclear membranes, fixed and negatively stained	61 ± 8	74.3 ± 3.3

cryotome-sections of directly Freon-frozen oocytes appears nearly circular (see Scheer, 1970). Thus, it is likely that the dehydration process through ethanol or glycerol steps does not result in a shrinkage of the perinuclear cisterna but leads to a wrinkling of the nuclear envelope, thereby unaffecting the pore diameter or the pore frequency. Since the nuclear pore complexes apparently behave as skeleton-constituting structure, it is conceivable, in particular with the amphibian oocyte, that here cisternal shrinkage is prevented by the increased stabilization through the exceedingly high pore frequency: about 30% of the membrane surface area is occupied by pore complexes. On the other hand, however, it cannot be excluded that the non-sensitivity of the amphibian oocyte nuclear envelope might be due to a more "relaxed" in vivo state.

6. Some Conclusions and Remarks

The specific differences in the nuclear envelope structural data between the different cell systems, as have been described from thin section and negative staining techniques, can be demonstrated with the freeze-etch technique, as well. There is also an obvious difference in nuclear envelope behaviour from cell type to cell type in response to the different types of electron microscopic preparations (compare, e.g., the above given results from rat hepatocytes and from amphibian oocytes). On the other hand, the freeze-etch technique has revealed some basic common structural principles such as with the perinuclear cisternal architecture, the pore complex substructural details and the fracture planes and surfaces. It is interesting that certain structural pecularities of the nuclear pore complex in special cell types, found with the thin section and negative stain technique, such as are present, e.g., with the mature nucleated erythrocyte, i.e. lack of annulus and central granule material, could be confirmed in our freeze-etch study.

The fracture face aspects, which did not show any basic diversity between the different cell types as well as between inner and outer membrane, in our opinion augment the accumulating scepticism against the use of fracture aspects including the mode of distribution and the sizes of "particles" as morphological membrane markers. We regard this generalizing mode of membrane characterization all the more as not justified, since every freeze-etch electron microscopist can convince himself that such particles can be seen on diverse sorts of non-membranous surfaces as well (see, e.g., Fig. 42; compare also the micrographs published by Fluck et al., 1969; Watson and Remsen, 1969; Davy and Branton, 1970; Deamer et al., 1970).

Considering the differences in nuclear envelope freeze-etch appearance among the different cell systems it is on the other hand a significant result of our study that the characteristic fracture behaviour of nuclear membranes is basically the same as with quite different types of membranes including the plasma membranes, which are at the end of the "membrane differentiation sequence" as shown by the investigators at Purdue (Grove et al., 1968; Morre et al., 1971). For instance, the cleavage behaviour of the nuclear membrane is fully compatible with Branton's hypothesis and thus might indicate that the concept of a freeze-fracturing principle common to biomembranes in general might be justified.

Summary

The structure of the nuclear envelope was investigated in a comparative study of different plant and animal cell systems (rat hepatocytes, hen erythrocytes, amphibian oocytes, and the marine haptophycean alga *Pleurochrysis scherffelii*) using the freeze-etch technique. The observations obtained with this method are compared with those of electron microscopic studies using thin section and negative staining procedures.

When fractured in the nucleocytoplasmic direction the nuclear envelope generally reveals four aspects, namely two "fracture planes" distinct from each other and two "true surfaces" which are limited to narrow rims along the fracture steps. Mirror-image symmetrical aspects are observed when the fracture runs in the opposite direction. The "true surfaces" planes lie by 30–45 Å on top of the following "fracture planes". The results are summed up to an interpretative scheme of the splintering through the nuclear envelope and are compatible with the view that the freeze-etch technique preferentially exposes aspects of the membrane interior (Branton, 1966). Inner and outer nuclear membranes are not significantly different in their freeze-etch appearance. With all the cell types studied, the nuclear pore complexes are suggested as being sites which tend to resist the membrane cleaving processes and thus frequently bring about localized changes of the fracture line. The diverse possibilities of how a pore complex can behave in the membrane fracturing are comprised in schemes. The freeze-etch appearance of the pore complex substructural constituents is described. The distribution pattern and the diameters of the pores have been evaluated. The measurements indicate that interruptions within the nuclear envelope as seen with the freeze-etch procedure do not necessarily represent fractured nuclear pores but might also reflect other structural situations including the production of "pore-corresponding holes" with diameters more or less larger than the true diameter of the pore itself. Structural data (pore frequency, pore diameter) of the frozen-etched cells were compared with those from sections through whole cells, isolated nuclei and isolated nuclear membranes after the usual dehydration treatments and from negative staining preparations of isolated nuclear envelope fragments, as well as with the corresponding data of frozen-etched isolated nuclei or nuclear membranes. The amphibian oocytes do not show significant differences in relation to the different procedures whereas such are well pronounced with, e.g., rat liver cells. The divergent results are discussed along the hypothesis of nuclear envelope shrinkage during the fragmentation and dehydration procedures.

Note Added in Proof. Since the acceptance of the present article (14. April 1971) a paper by Plattner (1971) has appeared in which the reality of the membranous "freeze-etch particles" is generally questioned on the basis on a comparative study using different cryofixation techniques: "In summary, I want to emphasize, that membrane bound "granules" in freeze-etch preparations might to a certain extent be segregation artifacts."

Acknowledgement. We gratefully acknowledge the skilful technical assistance of Miss Sigrid Krien and Miss Marianne Winter as well as the intense discussions with Drs. H. Falk and R. M. Brown (University of North Carolina, Chapel Hill, U.S.A.). To the latter we are also indebted for providing the cultures of Pleurochrysis. We also thank Dipl. Biol. C. E. Reilly for correcting the manuscript and Mr. V. Speth for the initial instructions at the freeze-etch apparatus. The work was supported by the Deutsche Forschungsgemeinschaft (grant No. Fr 308/4).

References

Accola, P.: Isolierung von Zellkernen aus Zwiebelwurzeln. Ber. schweiz. bot. Ges. **70,** 352–394 (1960).

Allen, J. V., Hess, W. M.: Ultrastructure of Tilletia caries teliospores as revealed by freeze-etching. J. Cell Biol. **43,** 4a (1969).

Anderson, N. G., Wilbur, K. M.: Studies on isolated cell components. IV. The effect of various solutions on the isolated rat liver nucleus. J. gen. Physiol. **35,** 781–790 (1952).

Arntzen, C. J., Dilley, R. A., Crane, F. L.: A comparisation of chloroplast membrane surfaces visualized by freeze-etch and negative staining techniques; and ultrastructural characterization of membrane fractions obtained from digitonin treated spinach chloroplasts. J. Cell Biol. **43,** 16–31 (1969).

Bachmann, L., Abermann, R., Zingsheim, H. P.: Hochauflösende Gefrierätzung. Histochemie **20,** 133–142 (1969).

Bahr, G. F., Beermann, W.: The fine structure of the nuclear membrane in the larval salivary gland and midgut of Chironomus. Exp. Cell Res. **6,** 519–522 (1954).

Bajer, A., Mole-Bajer, J.: Formation of spindle fibers, kinetochore orientation and behavior of the nuclear envelope during mitosis in endosperm — Fine structural and in vivo studies. Chromosoma (Berl.) **27,** 448–484 (1969).

Barnes, B. G., Davies, J. M.: The structure of nuclear pores in mammalian tissue. J. Ultrastruct. Res. **3,** 131–146 (1959).

Bauer, H.: Interpretation of frozen-fractured membranes of Lipomyces lipofer. J. Bact. **96,** 853–854 (1968).

Bayer, M. E., Remsen, C. C.: Structure of E. coli after freeze-etching. J. Bact. **101,** 304–313 (1970).

Beams, H. W., Mueller, S.: Effects of ultracentrifugation on the interphase nucleus of somatic cells with special reference to the nuclear envelope-chromatin relationship. Z. Zellforsch. **108,** 297–308 (1970).

Bererhi, A., Malkani, K.: Etude des cellules HeLa en culture par le cryodecapage. J. Ultrastruct. Res. **32,** 23–31 (1970).

Berezney, R., Funk, L. K., Crane, F. L.: The isolation of nuclear membrane from large-scale preparation of bovine liver nuclei. Biochim. biophys. Acta (Amst.) **203,** 531–546 (1970).

— — — Electron transport in mammalian nuclei. II. Oxidative enzymes in a large-scale preparation of bovine liver nuclei. Biochim. biophys. Acta (Amst.) **223,** 61–70 (1970b).

Bertaud, W. S., Rayns, D. G., Simpson, F. O.: Freeze-etch studies on fish skeletal muscle. J. Cell Sci. **6,** 537–557 (1970).

Betel, I.: The endogenous substrate for nuclear oxidative phosphorylation. Arch. Biochem. Biophys. **184**, 271–274 (1969).

Bischoff, A., Moor, H.: Ultrastructural differences between the myelin sheats of peripheral nerve fibres and CNS white matter. Z. Zellforsch. **81**, 303–310 (1967).

Bishop, W. R.: Methodology of rapid deep freeze cleavage replication of mammalian tissues and cells. Balzers Fachbericht Nr. 24 (1969).

Bracker, C. H., Grove, S. N.: Surface structure on outer mitochondrial membranes of Pythium ultimum. Cytobiol. **3**, 229–239 (1971).

Branton, D.: Fracture faces of frozen membranes. Proc. nat. Acad. Sci. (Wash.) **55**, 1048–1056 (1966).

— Fracture faces of frozen myelin. Exp. Cell Res. **45**, 703–707 (1967).

— Membrane structure. Ann. Rev. Plant Physiol. **20**, 209–238 (1969).

— Moor, H.: Fine structure in freeze-etched Allium cepa L. root tips. J. Ultrastruct. Res. **11**, 401–411 (1964).

— Park, R. B.: Subunits in chlorplast lamellae. J. Ultrastruct. Res. **19**, 283–303 (1967).

— Southworth, D.: Fracture faces of frozen Chlorella and Saccharomyces cells. Exp. Cell Res. **47**, 648–653 (1967).

Brettschneider, L. H.: The electron-microscopic investigation of tissue sections. Int. Rev. Cytol. 1, 305–322 (1952).

Brown, R. M., Franke, W. W.: A microtubular crystal associated with the Golgi field of Pleurochrysis scherffelii. Planta (Berl.) **96**, 354–363 (1971).

— Franke, W. W., Kleinig, H., Falk, H., Sitte, P.: Scale formation in Chrysophycean algae. I. Cellulosic and non-cellulosic wall components made by the Golgi apparatus. J. Cell Biol. **45**, 246–271 (1970).

Bullivant, S., Ames, A.: A simple freeze-fracture replication method for electron micr oscopy J. Cell Biol. **29**, 435–459 (1966).

Buttrose, M. S.: Ultrastructure of Barley aleurone cells as shown by freeze-etching. Planta (Berl.) **96**, 13–26 (1971).

Callan, H. G., Lloyd, L.: Lampbrush chromosomes of crested newts Triturus cristatus (Laurenti). Phil. Trans. roy. Soc. London B **243**, 135–219 (1960).

— Tomlin, S. G.: Experimental studies on amphibian oocyte nuclei by means of the electron microscope. I. Investigation of the structure of the nuclear membrane. Proc. roy. Soc. B **137**, 367–378 (1970).

Chalcroft, J. P., Bullivant, S.: An interpretation of liver cell membrane and junction structure based on observations of freeze-fracture replicas of both sides of the fracture. J. Cell Biol. **47**, 49–60 (1970).

Clark, A. W., Branton, D.: Fracture faces in frozen segments from the guinea pig retina. Z. Zellforsch. **91**, 586–603 (1968).

Clerot, J. C.: Mise en évidence par cytochimie ultrastructurale de lémission de protéines par le noyau d'auxocytes de batraciens. J. Microscopie **7**, 973–992 (1968).

Comes, P., Franke, W. W.: Composition, structure and function of the HeLa cell nuclear envelope. Z. Zellforsch. **107**, 240–248 (1970).

Comings, D. E., Okada, T. A.: Association of chromatin fibres with the annuli of the nuclear membrane. Exp. Cell Res. **62**, 293–302 (1970a).

— — Association of nuclear membrane fragments with metaphase and anaphase chromosomes as observed by whole mount electron microscopy. Exp. Cell Res. **63**, 62–68 (1970b).

Conover, T. E.: On the occurence of respiratory components in calf thymus nuclei. I. Low temperature spectra. Arch. Biochem. Biophys. **136**, 541–550 (1970a).

— On the occurence of respiratory components in calf thymus nuclei. II. Cytochrome oxidase activity. Arch. Biochem. Biophys. **136**, 551–562 (1970b).

Daniels, E. W., McNiff, J. M., Ekberg, D. R.: Nucleopores of the giant amoeba, Pelomyxa carolinensis. Z. Zellforsch. **98**, 357–363 (1969).

DaSilva, P. P., Branton, D.: Membrane splitting in freeze-etching. J. Cell Biol. **45**, 598–605 (1970).

— Douglas, S. D., Branton, D.: Location of A_1 antigens on the human erythrocyte membrane. J. Cell Biol. **47**, 159 A (1970).

Davies, H. G.: Electron-microscope observations on the organization of heterochromatin in certain cells. J. Cell Sci. 3, 129–150 (1968).

Davy, J. G., Branton, D.: Subliming ice surfaces: freeze-etch electron microscopy. Science 168, 1216–1218 (1970).

Deamer, D. W., Leonard, R., Tardieu, A., Branton, D.: Lamellar and hexagonal lipid phases visualized by freeze-etching. Biochim. biophys. Acta (Amst.) 219, 47–60 (1970).

Deumling, B., Franke, W. W.: Nuclear membranes from mammalian liver. VI. On the topology of nuclear DNA replicase activity. In preparation (1971).

DeZoeten, G. A., Gaard, G.: Possibilities for inter- and intracellular translocation of some icosahedral plant viruses. J. Cell Biol. 40, 814–823 (1969).

DuPraw, E. I.: The organization of nuclei and chromosomes in honeybee embryonic cells. Proc. nat. Acad. Sci. (Wash.) 53, 161–168 (1965).

Easterbrook, K. B., Rozee, K. R.: The ultrastructure of Rheovirus inclusion: A freeze-etching study. J. Ultrastruct. Res. 34, 303–315 (1971).

Engstrom, L., Branton, D.: Observations on freeze-etched erythrocyte membranes. J. Cell Biol. 39, 40A (1968).

Everid, A. C., Small, J. V., Davies, H. G.: Electron-microscope observations on the structure of condensed chromatin: Evidence for orderly arrays of unit threads on the surface of chicken erythrocyte nuclei. J. Cell Sci. 7, 35–48 (1970).

Fill, A., Branton, D.: Changes in the plasma membrane of E. coli during magnesium starvation. J. Bact. 98, 1320–1327 (1969).

Fineran, B. A.: Organization of the tonoplast in frozen-etched root tips. J. Ultrastruct. Res. 33, 574–586 (1970a).

— The effects of various pre-treatments on the freeze-etching of root tips. J. Microscopy 92, 85–97 (1970b).

Fisher, H. W., Cooper, T. W.: Electron microscope observations on the nuclear pores of HeLa cells. Exp. Cell Res. 48, 620–622 (1967).

Fluck, D. J., Henson, A. F., Chapman, D.: The structure of dilute lecithin-water systems revealed by freeze-etching and electron microscopy. J. Ultrastruct. Res. 29, 416–429 (1969).

Franke, W. W.: Isolated nuclear membranes. J. Cell Biol. 31, 619–623 (1966).

— Zur Feinstruktur isolierter Kernmembranen aus tierischen Zellen. Z. Zellforsch. 80, 585–593 (1967).

— Universality of the nuclear pore complex structure. Z. Zellforsch. 105, 405–429 (1970).

— Strukturen und Funktionen der Zellkernmembran: Zur Nukleinsäure-Interaktion. Cytobiol., in press (1971).

— Deumling, B., Ermen, B., Jarasch, E. D., Kleinig, H.: Nuclear membranes from mammalian liver. I. Isolation procedures and general characterisation. J. Cell Biol. 46, 379–395 (1970).

— Falk, H.: Appearance of nuclear pore complexes after Bernhard's staining procedure. Histochemie 24, 266–278 (1970).

— Kartenbeck, J.: Structures of nuclear membranes isolated from brain cells. Experientia (Basel) 25, 306–308 (1969).

— — Deumling, B.: Nuclear pore flow rates of ribonucleic acids in the mature rat hepatocyte. Experientia (Basel) 27, 372–373 (1971).

— Krien, S., Brown, R. M.: Simultaneous glutaraldehyde-osmium tetroxide fixation with postosmication. Histochemie 19, 162–164 (1969).

— Scheer, U.: The ultrastructure of the nuclear envelope of the amphibian oocyte. I. The mature oocyte. J. Ultrastruct. Res. 30, 288–316 (1970a).

— — The ultrastructure of the nuclear envelope of amphibian oocytes: a reinvestigation. II. The immature oocyte and dynamic aspects. J. Ultrastruct. Res. 30, 317–327 (1970b).

— Schinko, W.: Nuclear shape in muscle cells. J. Cell Biol. 42, 326–331 (1969).

Frey-Wyssling, A., Mühlethaler, K.: Ultrastructural plant cytology, p. 182–189. Amsterdam-London-New York: Elsevier Publ. Co. 1965.

Friederici, H. H. R.: The surface structure of some renal cell membranes. Lab. Invest. 21, 459–471 (1969).

Gall, J. G.: Observations on the nuclear membrane with the electron microscope. Exp. Cell Res. 7, 197–200 (1954).

Gall, J. G.: Small granules in amphibian oocyte nucleus and their relationship to RNA. J. biophys. biochem. Cytol. **2**, Suppl., 393–396 (1956).
— Octagonal nuclear pores. J. Cell Biol. **32**, 391–399 (1967).
Giesbrecht, P.: Über die Tertiärstruktur der DNS in den Chromosomen lebender Zellen. Z. Naturforsch. **20b**, 927–928 (1965).
— Drews, G.: Über die Organisation und die makromolekulare Architektur der Thylakoide „lebender" Bakterien. Arch. Mikrobiol. **54**, 297–330 (1966).
Gilula, N. B., Branton, D., Satir, P.: The septate junction: A structural basis for intercellular coupling. Proc. nat. Acad. Sci. (Wash.) **67**, 213–220 (1970).
Gool, A. van, Meyer, J., Lambert, R.: The fine structure of frozen etched Fusanum conidospores. J. Microscopie **9**, 653–660 (1970).
Gouranton, J.: L'envelope nucléaire. Ann. Biol. **8**, 385–409 (1969).
Grove, S. N., Bracker, C. E., Morre, D. J.: Cytomembrane differentiation in the endoplasmatic reticulum-Golgi apparatus-vesicle complex. Science **161**, 171–173 (1968).
Hartmann, J. F.: An electron optical study of sections of the central nervous system. J. comp. Neurol. **99**, 201–249 (1953).
Helander, H. F.: Surface topography of ultramicrotome sections. J. Ultrastruct. Res. **29**, 373–382 (1969).
Hess, W. M.: Ultrastructural comparisons of fungus hyphal cells using frozen-etched replicas and thin sections of the fungus Pyrenochaeta terrestis. Canad. J. Microbiol. **14**, 203–210 (1968).
Holt, S. C., Stern, A. L.: The effect of 3-(3.4-dichlorphenyl)-1.1-dimethylurea on chloroplast development and maintenance in Euglena gracilis. I. Ultrastructural characterization of light grown cells by the techniques of thin sectioning and freeze-etching. Plant Physiol. **45**, 475–483 (1970).
Jackson, V., Earnhardt, J., Chalkley, R.: A DNA-lipid protein containing material isolated from calf thymus nuclear chromatin. Biochem. biophys. Res. Commun. **33**, 253–259 (1968).
Jarasch, E.-D.: Enzymaktivitäten von isolierten Kernmembranen aus Säugetierleber. Diplomarbeit, Universität Freiburg i. Br., p. 1–41 (1969).
— Kartenbeck, J., Franke, W. W.: Nuclear membranes from mammalian liver. V. The question of the glucose-6-phosphatase activity. Manuscript in preparation (1971).
Jost, M., Jones, D. D.: Morphological parameters and macromolecular organization of gas vacuole membranes of Microcystis aerigunosa Kuetz. emend. Elenkin. Canad. J. Microbiol. **16**, 159–164 (1970).
Kashnig, D. M., Kasper, B. C.: Isolation, morphology and composition of the nuclear membrane from rat liver. J. biol. Chem. **244**, 3786–3792 (1969).
Kasper, C. B.: Biochemical distinctions between the nuclear and microsomal membranes from rat hepatocytes. J. biol. Chem. **246**, 577–581 (1971).
Kautz, J., DeMarsh, Q. B.: The fine structure of the nuclear membrane in cells from the chick embryo: on the nature of the so-called "pores" in the nuclear membrane. Exp. Cell Res. **8**, 394–396 (1955).
Kaye, J. S.: The ultrastructure of chromatin in nuclei of interphase cells in spermatids. In: Handbook of molecular cytology, ed. by A. Lima de Faria, p. 361–380. Amsterdam and London: North Holland Publ. Co. 1969.
Keenan, F. W., Berezney, R., Funk, L., Crane, F. L.: Lipid composition of nuclear membranes isolated from bovine liver. Biochim. biophys. Acta (Amst.) **203**, 547–554 (1970).
Keyhani, E.: Etude au microscope électronique de la structure des mégacaryocytes de cobaye par la technique de cryodécapage. Comparison avec la technique des coupes. J. Microscopie **9**, 63–74 (1970).
— Kriz, J.: Ultrastructure de la membrane mitochondriale. Etude par coloration négative et cryodécapage. C. R. Acad. Sci. (Paris) **268**, 1643 (1969).
Kleinig, H.: Nuclear membranes from mammalian liver. II. Lipid composition. J. Cell Biol. **46**, 396–402 (1970).
— Zentgraf, H., Comes, P., Stadler, J.: Nuclear membranes and plasma membranes from hen erythrocytes. II. Lipid composition. J. biol. Chem., **24b**, 2996–3000 (1971).
Koehler, J. K.: Nuclear structure in bull spermatozoa as revealed by freeze-etching. VI. Int. Congr. Electr. Micr., Kyoto, Vol. II, 641–642 (1966).

Koehler, J. K.: The technique and application of freeze-etching in ultrastructure research. Advanc. biol. med. Phys. 12, 1–20 (1968a).
— Freeze-etching observations on nucleated erythrocytes with special reference to the nuclear and plasma membranes. Z. Zellforsch. 85, 1–17 (1968b).
— A freeze-etching study of rabbit spermatozoa with particular reference to head structures. J. Ultrastruct. Res. 33, 598–614 (1970).
Kouri, J., Finlayand, C., Stark, G.: Study of rabbit alveolar macrophage by freeze etching. J. Microscopie 9, 177–184 (1970).
Kuzmina, S. N., Zbarsky, J. B., Monakhov, N. K., Gaitzkhoki, V. S., Neifakh, S. A.: Respiration in isolated rat liver nuclear envelopes. Federation of European Biochemical Societies, Letters (Amsterdam) 5, 34–36 (1969).
Leak, L. V.: Ultrastructure of proximal tubule cells in mouse kidney as revealed by freeze-etching. J. Ultrastruct. Res. 25, 253–270 (1968).
— Fractured surfaces of myocardial cells. J. Ultrastruct. Res. 31, 76–94 (1970).
Markham, R., Frey, S., Hills, G. J.: Methods for the enhancement of image detail and accentuation of structure in electron microscopy. Virology 20, 88–102 (1963).
Matile, P.: Lysosomes of root tip cells in corn seedlings. Planta (Berl.) 79, 181–196 (1968).
— Moor, H.: Vacuolation: Origin and development of the lysosomal apparatus in root-tip cells. Planta (Berl.) 80, 159–175 (1968).
Maul, G. G.: The relationship of nuclear pores to chromatin. J. Cell Biol. 47, 132A (1970).
McNutt, N., Weinstein, R. S.: The ultrastructure of the nexus. A correlated thin-section and freeze-cleave study. J. Cell Biol. 47, 666–688 (1970).
Mentre, P.: Présence d'acide ribonucléique dans l'anneau osmiophile et le granule central des pores nucléaires. J. Microscopie 8, 51–68 (1969).
Meyer, H. W., Winkelmann, H.: Die Gefrierätzung und die Struktur biologischer Membranen. Protoplasma (Wien) 68, 253–270 (1969).
— — Nachweis der Membranspaltung bei der Gefrierätzpräparation an Erythrozyten-ghosts und die Beeinflussung der Membranstruktur durch Harnstoff. Protoplasma (Wien) 70, 233–246 (1970).
Mizuno, N. S., Stoops, C. E., Sinha, A. A.: DNA synthesis associated with the inner membrane of the nuclear envelope. Nature New Biol. 229, 22–24 (1971).
Monroe, J. H., Schidlovsky, G., Chandra, S.: Membrane pores and herpesvirus-type particles in negatively stained whole cells. J. Ultrastruct. Res. 21, 134–144 (1967).
Moor, H.: Die Gefrierfixation lebender Zellen und ihre Anwendung in der Elektronenmikroskopie. Z. Zellforsch. 62, 546–580 (1964).
— Der Feinbau der Mikrotubuli in Hefe nach Gefrierätzung. Protoplasma (Wien) 64, 89–103 (1967).
— Freeze-etching. Int. Rev. Cytol. 25, 391–412 (1969a).
— Beitrag der Gefrierätzmethode zur Aufklärung von Struktur und Funktion der Biomembranen. Ber. dtsch. bot. Ges. 82, 385–396 (1969b).
— Mühlethaler, K.: Fine structure in frozen-etched yeast cells. J. Cell Biol. 17, 609–628 (1963).
— — Waldner, H., Frey-Wyssling, A.: A new freezing-ultramicrotome. J. biophys. biochem. Cytol. 10, 1–13 (1961).
— Pfenninger, K., Akert, K.: Synaptic vesicles in electron micrographs of freeze-etched nerve terminals. Science 164, 1405–1407 (1969).
Morre, D. J., Cheetham, R., Yunghaus, W.: Biochemical characterization of a Golgi apparatus-rich cell fraction isolated from rat liver. J. Cell Biol. 39, 96a (1968).
— Merlin, L. M., Keenan, T. W.: Localization of glycosyl transferase activities in a Golgi apparatus-rich fraction isolated from rat liver. Biochem. biophys. Res. Commun. 37, 813–819 (1969).
— Mollenhauer, H. H., Bracker, C. E.: Origin and continuity of Golgi apparatus. In: Results and problems in cell differentiation, vol. 2, origin and continuity of cell organelles, ed. by J. Reinert and H. Ursprung, p. 82–126. Berlin-Heidelberg-New York: Springer 1971.
Moule, Y.: In Structure and function of the endoplasmic reticulum in animal cells, ed. by F. C. Grand, p. 1–12. New York: Academic Press 1968.

Müller, H. O.: Die Ausmessung übermikroskopischer Objekte in ihrer Tiefe. Kolloid-Z. **99**, 6–8 (1942).

Mukherjee, T. M., Staehelin, L. A.: The fine-structural organization of the brush border of intestinal epithelial cells. J. Cell Sci. 8, 573–599 (1971).

Nanninga, N.: Ultrastructure of the cell envelope of E. coli B after freeze-etching. J. Bact. **101**, 297–303 (1970).

Neushul, M.: A freeze-etching study of the red alga Porphyridium. Amer. J. Bot. **57**, 1231–1239 (1970).

Nickel, E., Grieshaber, E.: Elektronenmikroskopische Darstellung der Muskelkapillaren im Gefrierätzbild. Z. Zellforsch. **95**, 445–461 (1969).

Northcote, D. H.: Structure and function of plant-cell membranes. Brit. med. Bull. **24**, 107–112 (1968).

— Lewis, D. R.: Freeze-etched surfaces of membranes and organelles in the cells of pea root tip. J. Cell Sci. **3**, 199–206 (1968).

O'Brien, J. S.: Cell membranes-composition: structure: function. J. theor. Biol. **15**, 307–324 (1967).

Ormerod, M. G., Lehmann, A. R.: The release of high molecular weight DNA from a mammalian cell (L_{517} 8 y). Attachment of the DNA to the nuclear membrane. Biochim. biophys. Acta (Amst.) **228**, 331–343 (1971).

Park, R. B., Pfeifhofer, A. O.: Ultrastructural observations on deep-etched thylakoids. J. Cell Sci. **5**, 299–311 (1969 a).

— — The effect of ethylenediaminetetraacetate washing on the structure of spinach thylakoids. J. Cell Sci. **5**, 313–319 (1969 b).

Plattner, H.: Bull spermaotzoa: a re-investigation by freeze-etching using widely different cryofixation procedures. J. Submicr. Cytol. **3**, 19–32 (1971).

— Winkler, H., Hörtnagl, H., Pfaller, W.: A study of the adrenal medulla and its subcellular organelles by the freeze-etching method. J. Ultrastruct. Res. 28, 191–202 (1969).

Pitot, H. C., Sladek, N., Ragland, W., Murray, R. K., Mayer, G., Soling, H. D., Jost, J. P.: A possible role of the endoplasmic reticulum in the regulation of genetic expression. The membron concept. In: Microsomes and drug oxidation, ed. by J. R. Gilette, A. H. Conney, G. J. Cosmides, R. W. Estabrook, J. R. Fouts, G. J. Mannering, p. 59–79. New York and London: Academic Press 1969.

Rayns, D. G., Simpson, F. O., Bertaud, W. S.: Surface features of striated muscle. I. Guinea pig cardiac muscle. J. Cell Sci. **3**, 467–474 (1968).

— — — Surface features of striated muscle. II. Guinea pig skeletal muscle. J. Cell Sci. **3**, 475–482 (1968).

Reilly, C. E.: Isolierte Kernmembranen aus Kalbsthymus. Diplomarbeit, Universität Freiburg i. Br. 1971.

Reith, A., Oftebro, R.: The structure of HeLa cells after treatment with glycerol as revealed by freeze-etching and electron microscopic methods. J. Ultrastruct. Res. in press (1971).

Remsen, C. C.: Fine structure of the mesosome and nucleoid in frozen-etched Bacillus subtilis. Arch. Mikrobiol. **61**, 40–47 (1968).

— Lundgren, D. G.: Electron microscopy of the cell envelope of Ferrobacillus ferrooxidans prepared by freeze-etching and chemical fixation techniques. J. Bact. **92**, 1765–1771 (1966).

— Valois, F. W., Watson, S. W.: Fine structure of cytomembranes of Nitrosocystis oceanus. J. Bact. **94**, 422–433 (1967).

Richter, H., Sleytr, U.: Fettextraktion bei −78° C: Nachweis im Gefrierätzbild. Z. Naturforsch. **26** b, 470–473 (1971).

Roberts, K., Northcote, D. H.: Structure of the nuclear pore in higher plants. Nature (Lond.) **228**, 385–386 (1970).

Rupec, M., Sekeris, K.: Cytochromoxidase in Zellkernen von Kalbsthymocyten. Cytobiol., in press (1971).

Ruska, C., Ruska, H.: Kompartimentierung und Membran von Herzmuskel-Mitochondrien in Darstellungen durch die Gefrierätztechnik. Z. Zellforsch. **97**, 298–312 (1969).

Ryser, U.: Die Ultrastruktur der Mitosekerne in den Plasmodien von Physarum polycephalum. Z. Zellforsch. **110**, 108–130 (1970).

Satir, P., Gilula, N. B.: Freeze-etch of cilia. J. Cell Biol. **47**, 179a (1970).

Scheer, U.: Strukturen und Funktionen der Porenkomplexe in der Amphibien-Eizelle. Dissertation (University of Freiburg i. Br., Germany), p. 1–174 (1970).

— On the chemical nature of the pore complex material of amphibian oocytes. Submitted to J. Cell Biol. (1971).

— Franke, W. W.: Negative staining and adenosine triphosphatase activity of annulate lamellae of newt oocytes. J. Cell Biol. **42**, 519–533 (1969).

Schinko, W.: Untersuchungen an isolierten Zellkernen aus Rattenskelettmuskulatur. Staatsexamensarbeit, Universität Freiburg i. Br., p. 1–36 (1970).

Schwelitz, F. D., Evans, W. R., Mollenhauer, H. H., Dilley, R. A.: The fine structure of the pellicle of Euglena gracilis as revealed by freeze-etching. Protoplasma (Wien) **69**, 341–349 (1970).

Silverman, L., Schreiner, B., Glick, D.: Measurement of thickness within sections by quantitative electron microscopy. J. Cell Biol. **40**, 768–772 (1969).

Sitte, H.: Volumen und Flächenbestimmung nach Schnitt- und Abdruckbildern. Seminar 2470 „Grundlagen der Elektronenmikroskopie" der Techn. Akademie Esslingen (1964).

Sitte, P.: Biomembranen: Struktur und Funktion. Ber. dtsch. bot. Ges. **82**, 329–383 (1969).

Sjöstrand, F. S.: A comparison of plasma membrane, cytomembranes, and mitochondrial membrane elements with respect to ultrastructural features. J. Ultrastruct. Res. **9**, 561–580 (1963).

— The limit of section thickness. In: Electron microscopy of cells and tissue, vol. I, Instrumentation and techniques, p. 281–287. New York and London: Academic Press 1967.

— Ultrastructure and function of cellular membranes. In: The membranes, ed. by A. J. Dalton and F. Haguenau, p. 151–210. New York and London: Academic Press 1968.

Sleyter, U.: Die Gefrierätzung korrespondierender Bruchhälften: ein neuer Weg zur Aufklärung von Membranstrukturen. Protoplasma (Wien) **70**, 101–117 (1970).

Smith, S. J., Adams, H. R., Smetana, K., Busch, H.: Isolation of the outer layer of the nuclear envelope. Exp. Cell Res. **55**, 185–197 (1969).

Speth, V., Wunderlich, F.: The macronuclear envelope of Tetrahymena pyriformis GL in different physiological states. III. Appearance of freeze-etched nuclear pore complexes. J. Cell Biol. **47**, 772–777 (1970).

Spycher, M. A.: Intercellular adhesions. An electron microscope study on freeze-etched rat hepatocytes. Z. Zellforsch. **111**, 64–74 (1970).

Stadler, J., Kleinig, H.: Nuclear membranes of mammalian liver. III. Fatty acids. Biochim. biophys. Acta (Amst.) **233**, 315–319 (1971).

Staehelin, L. A.: The interpretation of freeze-etched artificial and biological membranes. J. Ultrastruct. Res. **22**, 326–347 (1968a).

— Ultrastructural changes of the plasmalemma and the cell wall during the life cycle of Cyanidium caldarium. Proc. roy. Soc. B **171**, 249–259 (1968b).

— Kiermayer, O.: Membrane differentiation in the Golgi complex of Micrasterias denticulata Breb. J. Cell Sci. **7**, 787–492 (1970).

— Mukherjee, T. M., Williams, A. W.: Freeze-etch appearance of tight junctions in the epithelium of small and large intestine of mice. Protoplasma (Wien) **67**, 165–184 (1969).

Steere, R. L.: Electron microscopy of structural detail in frozen biological specimens. J. biophys. biochem. Cytol. **3**, 45–60 (1957).

Stevens, B. J., Andre, J.: The nuclear envelope. In: Handbook of molecular cytology, ed. by A. Lima-de-Faria, p. 837–871. Amsterdam-London: North-Holland Publ. Co. 1969.

Stoeckenius, W., Kunau, W. H.: Further characterization of particulate fractions from lysed cell envelopes of halobakterium Halobium and isolation of gas vacuole membranes. J. Cell Biol. **38**, 337–357 (1968).

Tauschel, H. D., Speth, V.: Der Geißelapparat von Rhodopseudomonas palustris. V. Darstellung des Polarorganells mit Hilfe der Gefrierätz-Methode. Cytobiol. **2**, 403–407 (1970).

Tillack, T. W., Marchesi, V. T.: Demonstration of the outer surface of freeze-etched red blood cell membranes. J. Cell Biol. **45**, 649–653 (1970).

Tillack. T. W., Carter, R., Razin, S.: Native and reformed mycoplasma Laid lawii membranes compared by freeze-etching. Biochim. biophys. Acta (Amst.) 219, 123–130 (1970 b).
— Scott, R. E., Marchesi, V. T.: Studies on the chemistry and function of the intramembraneous particles observed by freeze-etching of red blood cell membranes. J. Cell Biol. 47, 213 A (1970 a).
Ueda, K., Matsuura, T., Date, N.: The occurrence of cytochromes in the membranous structures of calf thymus nuclei. Biochem. biophys. Res. Commun. 34, 322–339 (1969).
Waaland, J. R., Branton, D.: Gas vacuole development in a blue-green alga. Science 163, 1339–1341 (1969).
Wallach, D. F. H.: Membrane lipids and the conformations of membrane proteins. J. gen. Physiol. 54, 3s–26c (1969).
Wartiovaara, J., Branton, D.: Visualization of ribosomes by freeze-etching. Exp. Cell Res. 61, 403–406 (1970).
Watson, M. L.: Pores in the mammalian nuclear membrane. Biochim. biophys. Acta (Amst.) 15, 475–479 (1954).
— The nuclear envelope. Its structure and relation to cytoplasmic membranes. J. biophys. biochem. Cytol. 1, 257–270 (1955).
— Further observations on the nuclear envelope of animal cells. J. biophys. biochem. Cytol. 6, 147–156 (1959).
— Remsen, C. C.: Macromolecular subunits in the walls of marine nitrifying bacteria. Science 163, 685–686 (1969).
— — Cell envelope of Nitrosocystis oceanus. J. Ultrastruct. res. 33, 148–160 (1970).
Wecke, J., Giesbrecht, P.: Freeze-etching of the nuclear membrane of dinoflagellates. Sept. Congrès International de Microscope Electronique, Grenoble, p. 233–234 (1970).
Weinstein, R. S., Bullivant, S.: The application of freeze-cleaving techniques to studies on red blood cell fine structure. Blood 29, 780–789 (1967).
— Clowes, A. W., McNutt, N. S.: Unit cleavage planes in frozen red cell membranes. Proc. Soc. exp. Biol. (N.Y.) 134, 1195–1198 (1970).
— Koo, V. M.: Penetration of red cell membranes by some membrane-associated particles. Proc. Soc. exp. Biol. (N.Y.) 128, 353–357 (1968).
Werz, G., Kellner, G.: Die Struktur des Golgi-Apparates bei gefrier-geätzten Dunaliella-Zellen. Protoplasma (Wien(69, 351–364 (1970).
Wisse, E.: An electron microscopic study of the fenestrated endothelial lining of rat liver sinusoids. J. Ultrastruct. Res. 31, 125–150 (1970).
Yoo, B. Y., Bayley, S. T.: The structure of pores in isolated nuclei. J. Ultrastruct. Res. 18, 651–660 (1967).
Zbarski, J. B., Perevoshchikova, K. A., Delektorskaya, L. N., Delektorsky, V. V.: Isolation and biochemical characteristics of the nuclear envelope. Nature (Lond.) 221, 257–259 (1969).
Zentgraf, H., Deumling, B., Franke, W. W.: Isolation and characterization of nuclei from bird erythrocytes. Exp. Cell Res. 56, 333–337 (1969).
— — Jarasch, E.-D., Franke, W. W.: Nuclear membranes and plasma membranes from hen erythrocytes. I. Isolation, characterization and comparison. J. biol. Chem. 246, 2986–2995 (1971).
— Morre, D. J., Franke, W. W.: freeze-fracture planes of isolated red liver Golgi apparatus. In preparation (1971).
— Scheer, U.: Freeze-etch appearance of amphibian egg yolk. Exp. Cell Res., submitted (1971).

Subject Index

Actomyosin 16
Algae 10
Amphibian oocytes 11, 42, 44
Annular subunits 31
Annulus material 29, 33, 44
Arrangement of pores 37

Bacterial cell 16
Blood 10
Blood lily 40

Cacodylate buffer 10
Cations 38
Central granule 31, 32, 44
Chromatin 39, 40
Chromosomes 11, 15
Chrysophyta 10
Cross-bridges 15
Cross fractures 11 ff., 18, 34

Dehydration 14, 44
Dictyosomal stacks 25
Dinoflagellatae 37
Direction of fracturing 18
— of shadowing 11
Distribution of pores
DNA 40

Endosperm 40
Epithelial cells 16
Equatorial plane 23
Erythrocytes 10, 18, 32, 35, 36, 38, 44

Fibrils 32, 33
Filamentous material 32
Fissure rim 23
Fixation procedures 10
Formaldehyde 10, 42
F-plane 17 ff.
Fracture face 18, 23, 34, 44
— holes 18, 23, 35
— plane 16 ff., 27, 44
— rim 18, 25
— scheme 17, 30, 34
Fragment size 40, 41, 42
Freon 22 10, 11

Glutaraldehyde 10, 38
Glycerol 10, 42, 44
Golgi apparatus 15

Heterochromatin 13, 14
High salt extraction 41

Inner fibrils 32
— ring 32
Intracisternal surface 23, 24
Isolated hen erythrocyte nuclear membranes 10
— nuclei 10, 11, 38, 40, 42
— nuclear envelopes 31, 37, 38

Junctions, gap 25
—, septate 25
—, tight 25

Kidney cell 15

Lampbrush oocytes 10, 42, 43
Lipid composition of membranes 25
Liquemin 10
Liquid nitrogen 11

Mammalian sperm 13
Markham's rotation technique 31
Membrane surface 16 ff., 25, 31
Metaphase chromosomes 11
Microfilament 16
Mitochondrial membrane 31
Mitosis 40
Musculature 16
Mussel gill epithelium 25
Myelin sheath 25
Myocardium nexus 25

Negative staining 10, 11, 13, 23, 31, 35, 45
Non-prime plane 23
Nuclear envelope 10, 11, 13, 14, 16, 17, 18, 24, 35, 36, 37, 42, 43
— membrane 10, 11, 13, 23, 31, 35, 45
— pore complex 11, 23, 24, 31, 34
— surface 11, 40
Nucleolus 11, 15
Nucleoplasm 18, 23
Nucleoprotein structure 15

Onion root tip 38
Oocytes 11, 42, 43, 44

Particles 11, 17, 18, 23, 24, 25, 27, 31, 44
Particle distribution 27
Perinuclear cisterna 11 f., 23, 25, 34, 42, 44
Pytium ultimum 31
Plasma membrane 11, 17, 18, 45